Making Sense of the New NHS White Paper

MARK BAKER

FOREWORD BY
CHRIS HAM

RADCLIFFE MEDICAL PRESS

© 1998 Mark Baker

Radcliffe Medical Press Ltd
18 Marcham Road, Abingdon, Oxon OX14 1AA

British Library Cataloguing in Publication Data

A catalogue record for this book is available from the British Library.

ISBN 1 85775 239 2

Library of Congress Cataloging-in-Publication Data is available.

Typeset by Acorn Bookwork, Salisbury, Wilts
Printed and bound by Biddles Ltd, Guildford and King's Lynn

Contents

Foreword

The Labour Government's plans for the future of the NHS and of public health, set out in the white and green papers, signal both continuity and change. Continuity is evident in the willingness of the new Government to borrow ideas from its predecessors where this suits its own purpose. Change is proposed in areas where Labour wishes to introduce its own thinking into the policy debate. The resulting 'third way' offers a synthesis of the old and the new.

Like the last major reforms to the NHS initiated by Margaret Thatcher in 1989, the Government's plans have been sketched in broad outline and much of the detail is missing. This means that NHS staff have been busy pouring over the white and green papers trying to interpret the Government's intentions and reading between the lines to anticipate what might happen next. It is in this context that Mark Baker's summary of and commentary on the Government's proposals should be read. As an experienced doctor and manager who has worked in a variety of senior roles, he is well placed to help readers make sense of what has been proposed and to work through the implications.

This book is at once a guide through the maze for those who are perplexed by the direction of travel and an initial exercise in anticipating the future. Professor Baker draws on his experience to identify the key elements in the policy documents that have been published and to offer a personal view on what they might mean in the longer term. While not everyone will agree with his analysis, it has the great merit of being written from a depth of understanding and experience of the issues. It therefore has a real feel of what life is like at the front line in a health service which often appears to be under siege. Professor Baker has an unusual capacity to relate government policy to what is happening on the ground, and to write about the wider implications in a way that can be understood by others. This book will not be the last analysis of New Labour and the NHS but it offers a useful starting point for practitioners and students of health policy.

Chris Ham
Health Services Management Centre
University of Birmingham
May 1998

Part 1

Introduction

The crisis

The state of the NHS posed a daunting challenge to the new Labour Government following its success in the general election of May 1997. Not only was the NHS deeply insolvent – trust and health authority combined book deficits estimated at up to £1 billion – but the morale of staff was low, even by NHS standards, and health service targets such as reduced waiting times and guaranteed admission for emergencies were being missed in vain pursuit of financial balance. Indeed, the triad of responsibilities for health authorities and NHS trusts – financial balance; containing waiting times to within NHS Charter and lower local limits; and guaranteeing local hospital care for emergencies – appeared to be beyond reach in many cases. It was clear to many observers that the hospital service had more beds than it could afford but not enough to meet demand. The internal market was generally perceived to have failed to deliver the benefits expected from markets, such as reduced costs, sensitivity to patient needs and higher quality of care. Fuelled by the Patient's Charter, public expectations of the NHS were rising and were further heightened by the prospect of a Labour administration after 18 years in opposition. The result of the British general election on 1 May 1997, led to an immediate and almost universal rise in the 'feel good' factor, reflected in opinion polls, the financial markets and public sector (including NHS) staff (with a few notable exceptions affected by Labour proposals such as GP fundholders). Meeting the expectations of the public and of NHS staff was always going to prove a tall order.

The politicians

The prospects of definitive early action by the new Government were initially hindered by the unexpected appointment of Frank Dobson as Secretary of State for Health. Although Mr Dobson had been an experienced and effective opposition health spokesman during the mid-1980s, he had not had contact with the NHS brief for a decade. The proposals of the Labour Party in opposition for the future of the NHS had to be reviewed in the context of a new political team and the severity of the pressures facing the NHS. The promised reduction in waiting times by 100 000 in the first year was hastily abandoned and added to the growing list of manifesto pledges whose timescale had slipped. Such was the acknowledgment of the difficulties facing Ministers that it was even rumoured that Dobson had been given the job in the expectation of failure and that he would be sacrificed in the first cabinet reshuffle. An alternative rumour was that the shadow spokesman, Chris Smith, had been regarded as too keen on spending (and was therefore sent to The Department of Culture where he could spend lottery players' money rather than taxpayers' money) and only an Old Labour hand like Dobson could deliver the pain that was necessary to restore reason to the NHS. However plausible, both of these hypotheses were no more than idle tittle tattle.

Funding

Early indications were encouraging. Responding to genuine fears of a winter crisis in hospitals, the Government released an additional £300 million, secured from savings in other departments, to ease pressures on health and social services during the second half of 1997/98. Although a significant proportion of these funds did not find their way into England's hospitals, £159 million was allocated to local health and social services, equivalent to more than 1% extra for the autumn and winter period and enough to avoid the winter miseries of the previous two years. This followed a statement from the Chancellor of the Exchequer offering additional resources for the NHS (and Education) in 1998/99 by raiding the Treasury's contingency fund. Unfortunately, these gains were also partly illusory as raised estimates of inflation and the hangover of phased 1997/98 pay awards accounted for half of the additional funding. The Government appeared to be clear that its priority was ensuring that emergencies were effectively treated in local hospitals and that other priorities – financial balance and waiting times – were of secondary importance. Later, either Ministers had second thoughts or civil servants anticipated what Ministers really meant; that is that all the imperatives remained in place but that managers were more likely to be sacked for failing to ensure that emergency demands were met. By January 1998, all three priorities had been restored as mandatory. Further additional funding of £50 million was found to protect hospital services in the most insolvent health authority areas, an action regarded in some quarters as rewarding failure. Nonetheless, it appeared that the Government was serious about keeping the NHS afloat, recognized the need to invest additional real resources and was genuine about retaining a comprehensive service. Indeed, by February 1998, waiting lists had re-emerged as a suitable case for treatment, and with an additional £500 million allocated in the March 1998 budget, every likelihood of becoming the benchmark for performance once again. Conversely, the phasing of the 1998/99 pay award for staff covered by the pay review bodies suggested no relaxation in public sector pay or funding in general. It has become clear that the priorities for the NHS in 1998/99 are to eradicate its financial deficit – so that the new money to be allocated thereafter delivers service benefits rather than merely reducing deficits – and to restore waiting lists to their March 1997 level. The NHS is unlikely to be a place for faint hearts in the immediate future.

Policy

Most new governments reorganize the NHS. It is not that there is any evidence that such changes are desirable, necessary or successful, merely that it is within the power of government to take such action. Thus, in almost every field of endeavour, the new Government issued proposals and/or legislation during its first six months, fuelled by the long years of opposition and by the comprehensive policy review undertaken after Tony Blair's election as leader. Rapid action followed in education, transport and, especially, devolution.

In the health service, however, we waited in vain for a prompt policy directive. Positive noises were made about public health and the Government's commitment to replace the internal market in the NHS was clearly signposted, as it had been before the election. The long promised reduction in management costs – normally referred to as 'bureaucracy' or 'red tape' – duly arrived but was little more than those cuts already agreed plus a postponement of the next (eighth) wave of GP fundholding. The anticipated public health Green Paper, expected in November 1997, was postponed; due to a classic error of organization, the launch meeting for chairs, chief executives and public health directors of health authorities went ahead on 17 November but Ministers had nothing new to say. The massive faux pas of the Formula One exclusion from the proposed ban on tobacco advertising had seriously wounded the Public Health Minister, Tessa Jowell, shortly before this meeting. The Health Action Zone initiative, which should. have followed the context setting of the public health policy, was duly published first. It was against this background that the long awaited White Paper was published in December 1997. The Green Paper on public health, *Our Healthier Nation*, was eventually published on 5 February 1998, presumably having been trashed at least once by 10 Downing Street and having rather lost its place as the front end of government action on health. The Government tells us that *Our Healthier Nation* provides the front end for all its health strategies and that it sets the scene for Health Action Zones, the role and purpose of the NHS and the accountability of health authorities. However, it was published last and while *The New NHS* was introduced by the Prime Minister, *Our Healthier Nation* was introduced by Health Ministers – the symbols are all wrong and the plot has been lost on the journey.

A White Paper

It is alleged that the White Paper was leaked in October 1997 and apparently authoritative reports of its contents were published in several newspapers. A strange period followed during which many civil servants assured NHS managers that the White Paper was completed and at the printers – and therefore by inference beyond amendment. Most senior civil servants claim to have written all or part of the White Paper and promises of its guaranteed publication by the end of the week or month (November) came from the very top of the office. Ministers went ballistic over the 'leaks' and instituted a siege-like security at all Department of Health offices, far tighter indeed than during the height of terrorist campaigns in London. To seasoned observers, the whole charade was hilarious as we all assumed that leaks come from Ministers' offices rather than from their staff. Although laughable, the siege mentality did affect the informal consultation which should have been in progress at this time. As a result, the dialogue with local authorities about their close involvement with NHS plans and the attendance of their representatives at health authority board meetings did not take place. There ensued a six-week interval during which we were assured that final touches were still being applied to the White Paper and some decisions had not yet been made. No one believed this. At last the great day came and all the pundits were proved wrong; the 'leaks' proved incomplete or inaccurate and it did appear that important changes had been introduced at a late stage, most particularly in terms of the future management of mental health and learning disabilities services.

Most modern political statements are characterized by stunts and slogans. Stunts create the mirage of action to make a difference while slogans are useful for electioneering. The title of the NHS White Paper, *The New NHS: modern, dependable*, is itself a slogan with no attempt to define its precise meaning throughout the document. The White Paper is structured into 10 chapters, all with a title, subheading and key themes, each of which is a freestanding slogan (*see* Box 1). The whole text is supported by margin sound-bites which are themselves intended to summarize in short slogans the thrust of Government policy (*see* Box 2). These phrases in the margins tell almost the whole story; they are the words which best define the Government's policies and priorities and may be the only bits of the document which were chosen by the politicians. I am, however, reliably informed that this White Paper has had a much stronger input from Ministers and particularly the Minister of State, Alan Milburn. The level of this political involvement is both a strength and a weakness; a strength in terms of political leadership, understanding and commitment; a weakness in the event of a promotion for the admirable Mr Milburn in the first cabinet reshuffle leaving the policy without political ownership within the Department of Health.

Box 1   Key themes

**A MODERN AND DEPENDABLE NHS
there when you need it**

- £1 billion from red tape into patient care

- NHS Direct – 24-hour nurse helpline

- NHS information superhighway

- Guaranteed fast-track cancer services

**A NEW START
what counts is what works**

- The third way

- Keeping what works

- Discarding what has failed

**DRIVING CHANGE IN THE NHS
quality and efficiency hand in hand**

- Raising quality standards

- Increasing efficiency
- Driving performance
- New roles and responsibilities

HEALTH AUTHORITIES
leading and shaping

- New focus on improving health
- New Health Improvement Programmes to shape local health care
- Lead strategic role for local NHS

PRIMARY CARE GROUPS
going with the grain

- Development of primary and community health care
- Family doctors and community nurses in the lead
- A spectrum of opportunities beyond fundholding

NHS TRUSTS
partnership and performance

- New role helping to plan local services
- Responsible for operational management
- New statutory duties for quality and partnership
- New emphasis on staff involvement

THE NATIONAL DIMENSION
a one nation NHS

- National leadership to support local development
- New National Institute for Clinical Excellence
- New Commission for Health Improvement

MEASURING PROGRESS
better every year

- New measures of NHS performance
- Action to tackle unacceptable service variations
- New national survey of patient experience

HOW THE MONEY WILL FLOW
from red tape to patient care

- Promoting quality and efficiency
- Stable funding
- Fair budgets
- £1 billion from bureaucracy

MAKING IT HAPPEN
rolling out change

- Building on what works
- Health Action Zones to blaze the trail
- A rolling programme of development

Box 2   Marginal soundbites

A MODERN AND DEPENDABLE NHS

- Prompt high-quality care
- Integrated care based on partnership and driven by performance
- More investment and better technology
- NHS Direct, a new 24-hour telephone line staffed by nurses
- Connecting every GP surgery and hospital to the NHS's own information superhighway

- Everyone with suspected cancer will be able to see a specialist within two weeks
- Tailoring the NHS to meet the needs of individual patients
- The health service is a strong and resilient organization
- We are committed to increasing spending on the NHS in real terms every year
- The health of the economy depends on the health of the NHS

A NEW START

- A new model for a new century
- Local doctors and nurses in the driving seat
- Excellence guaranteed to all patients
- The needs of patients not the needs of institutions will be at the heart of the new NHS
- Co-operation will replace competition
- Best practice available to patients wherever they live

DRIVING CHANGE IN THE NHS

- Raising standards and ensuring consistency
- A new statutory duty for quality
- Management costs will be capped
- The pursuit of quality and efficiency must go together if the NHS is to deliver the best for patients
- Leaner bodies with stronger powers (HAs)
- Commissioning services (PCGs)
- Providing services for patients (NHS trusts)
- Giving a national lead (DoH)

HEALTH AUTHORITIES

- Improving health and reducing inequalities
- They will act in partnership
- The first Health Improvement Programmes will be in place by April 1999
- More integrated health and social care services
- Targets that are measurable, published and deliver year-on-year improvement
- Communicating with local people and ensuring public involvement
- Fewer authorities covering larger areas
- Rewarding success

PRIMARY CARE GROUPS

- Primary care groups will grow out of the range of commissioning models that have developed in recent years
- Child health and rehabilitation services will particularly benefit
- The approach will be bottom-up and developmental
- Primary care trusts running community health services
- Deploying resources and savings to strengthen local services
- By cutting the number of commissioning bodies and scrapping both short-term contracts and individual case contracts, the new arrangements will also cut transaction costs and bureaucracy
- There will be accountability agreements between primary care groups and health authorities
- No barriers will be placed in the way of primary care groups which are making good progress
- Devolved commissioning will go hand-in-hand with greater equity
- Use their freedoms to improve primary and community care

- Primary care groups are where the future lies for GP fundholders

NHS TRUSTS

- Clear incentives available to help NHS trusts succeed

- Retain full responsibility for operational management

- Statutory duty for NHS trusts to work in partnership

- Twin guarantee of consistency and responsiveness

- A new duty for the quality of care

- When performance is not up to scratch in NHS trusts there will be rapid investigation and, when necessary, intervention

- Efficiency will be enhanced ... clinician-to-clinician partnership

- Longer-term service agreements to allow any savings to be redeployed

- Less bureaucracy and administration, but more good management

- A higher priority to human resource development

- Flexible, family-friendly, employment policies

- Taskforce on improving the involvement of frontline staff

- Greater involvement of clinical professionals

- The Government will make NHS trusts more open and accountable

- No management information to be 'commercial in confidence' between NHS bodies

THE NATIONAL DIMENSION

- National drive to improve quality and performance

- The Government will spread best practice and drive clinical and cost effectiveness

- Working with the professions to strengthen self-regulation
- Patients will get greater consistency in the availability and quality of services right across the NHS
- New coherence and prominence to information about clinical and cost effectiveness
- An independent guarantee that local systems to monitor, assure and improve clinical quality are in place
- The capacity for prompt and effective intervention
- Regional Offices will ensure local health services are working together to serve local people
- Supporting and developing local leaders
- A more systematic approach to guarantee fair access
- Clear quality control and assurance
- The NHS Executive will involve users and carers in its own work programme

MEASURING PROGRESS

- The way performance is measured and targets are set drives the way the NHS performs
- There will no longer be a narrow obsession with counting activity for the sake of it
- Greater benchmarking of performance
- A new NHS Charter
- The health service will measure itself against the aspirations and experience of its users
- First national survey will take place in 1998

HOW THE MONEY WILL FLOW

- NHS money will flow around the system to support quality and efficiency

- Encourage real efficiency as a means to a fair and high-quality service

- Raising spending on the NHS in real terms every year, with more of every pound going on patient care

- New mechanisms to distribute NHS cash more fairly

- The biggest new hospital building programme in the history of the NHS

- Freed from the constraints imposed by artificially distinct budget headings

- The NHS will ensure that all patients have proper access to the medicines they need

- A stable framework based on longer-term relationships

- The ECR system will be abolished

- A programme which requires NHS trusts to publish and benchmark their costs on a consistent basis

- Bearing down on costs to achieve best value

- This White Paper, by completing the abolition of the internal market, will release further resources from bureaucracy

- £1 billion will be freed up from bureaucracy for patient care

MAKING IT HAPPEN

- A clear direction for the NHS as a modern and dependable service

- The NHS getting better every year

- A rolling programme of modernization

- Health Action Zones will blaze the trail

- An NHS that responds to a changed and changing world

This style is not unusual and actually follows quite closely the manner of the previous Government's White Paper for NHS reform, *Working for Patients*. Like many previous reforms, *The New NHS* purports to support evolutionary change; indeed, the Labour Party in the run-up to the election had made much of its desire to avoid major reorganization. The NHS Chief Executive, Alan Langlands, is desperately trying to avoid the carnage and dysfunction of a wholesale restructuring which leads to most senior staff changing jobs. In practice, however, this White Paper heralds the most profound change in the structure of the NHS in its history. The Government may well be as sincere as Mr Langlands in its desire not to impose dysfunctional change on NHS structures unnecessarily, but it underestimates the pace and enthusiasm of NHS managers when reorganization is on the cards. Another proclaimed principle of the White Paper is the importance given to local views and bottom-up approaches. In practice, it is clear that this is a centralizing government and that control of these changes in the NHS is being strongly driven and managed from above. There is, however, a desire to persuade the people that they are empowered as shown in the devolution moves in Scotland and Wales and the elected mayor proposals for English cities. The Government has created for itself a risky paradox of being both centralizing and devolving at the same time. There are three sets of tensions in the approach to handling these paradoxes: the tension between vertical and lateral (horizontal) integration; between managed and entrepreneurial leadership; and between prescription (national) and flexibility (local). The desired outcome of these tensions is a balance in which the best of all worlds results.

What is it for?

While the headlines for the White Paper focus on replacing the internal market, merely a bureaucratic system for deciding how the money passes through the structure to where the costs are borne, it is the benefits for patients which should be the driving force. Government needs to decide what outcomes it seeks for users of its services and then to develop the structures and policies to deliver them. The benefits which the White Paper offers, sometimes indirectly, to patients are summarized in Box 3.

Box 3   Benefits for patients from *The New NHS*

- Better care for patients by integrating primary and community care and, perhaps, social care

- Releasing resources from hospital services by reducing variations in practice and thereby increasing efficiency, enabling waiting lists to be reduced

- Improving outcomes for patients by improving the effectiveness of clinical care, making health professionals more accountable for their clinical decisions

- Enhanced empowerment of patients, through easier access to information

---

The principal thrust of the whole document, and much else in the Government's approach to health and social care, is the integration of care outside hospital and between the community and hospital settings, despite all the obstacles. There is little doubt that there is much to gain by bringing together health and social services in the home. The biggest obstacles have been the political boundary between local government (which runs social services) and central government (which runs the NHS) and the imbalance in power of the various provider professions. It is an ambitious aspiration to achieve integration despite these. There remains confusion about whether the approach is to integrate commissioning of services or to integrate provision of care; since only the latter benefits patients directly, it should be the priority.

Funding or efficiency?

The Government has dismissed the idea that the NHS can only survive in its present form if it receives additional funding on a scale which would necessitate tax increases. It also rejects the possibility of formally restricting the scope of the NHS so that it ceases to be effectively comprehensive. These attitudes conflict with the feelings of most who work in the NHS and social services and those feelings find sympathy with some members of the public. The evidence must have been overwhelming to persuade Ministers to adopt a line which is so at odds with professional and public opinion. In the event, Ministers have been persuaded that there is sufficient waste in the hospital service to resource the existing shortfall and to improve services. The evidence to support this approach relies on observed variations in efficiency and the assumption that these variations can be eradicated in a way which releases resources. There is a precedent for this in the steep rise in day surgery and a narrowing of the variation between trusts. However, this strategy has two basic flaws: first, it will lead to major bed closures, never the most popular move politically; second, there are steeply rising pressures on hospital beds from rising emergency admissions and rising expectations. Only by closing beds and perhaps hospitals can sufficient resources be released to legitimize the Government's policy. Of course, the NHS will receive extra funds, but at present it looks as though they will be just enough to keep afloat.

Effectiveness too

The most ambitious, interesting and, probably, enduring strategy is in pursuit of effective clinical care and the emerging cloak of accountability for doctors and other health professionals under the title of 'clinical governance'. Both in this White Paper and in the Green Paper, *Our Healthier Nation*, effective health care is seen as the Holy Grail which everyone must pursue. This probably does the field a disservice in exaggerating its potential. There is no doubt that much can be achieved for patients by increasing the effectiveness of clinical care, but the lack of robust and reliable evidence for so many procedures and interventions will not reduce public and professional clamour for treatment regardless of the lack of evidence of effectiveness.

Competition, regulation and accountability

There is an interesting perspective on the growing management accountability being placed on managers and clinicians in this White Paper. In many respects, the NHS is becoming a regulated industry, like the former privatized utilities. Experience in most countries suggests that regulation does not work in terms of securing better services for consumers. In the UK, a combination of competition and naming and shaming poor performers appears to offer some advantage to customers in terms of quality of service and cost reductions and this Government is exceptionally keen to name and shame, for example in education and financial services. Competition has not worked too well in the NHS, probably due to the inflexibility of most services; it is likely therefore that the Government will want to adopt a name and shame strategy and this will start with the publication of hospital death rates. We all know that the data are rubbish but it will start people thinking about their outcomes and will, if nothing else, lead to the production of better and more reliable data. In any case, high-value benefits, such as improving services, are more likely to arise through collaboration rather than audit, i.e. through internal mechanisms not external control. Overseas observers describe regulated organizations in the UK as behaving like victims. I suspect that doctors in Britain will not submit to victimization and will fight this type of regulation all the way.

Working together

Another fundamental principle of the White Paper is the end of confrontation and the re-creation of an NHS family with unified planning systems, these including social services and the public. Having spent most of the last decade persuading NHS staff to behave competitively, it cannot be realistic to expect collectivism to emerge suddenly amongst health managers and professions and to universal acclaim. Of the existing players in the NHS market, only health authorities can have any reasonable claim to behave collaboratively and I know of many trusts who would dispute that.

Trusts and GPs are naturally competitive and members of Trust Boards have been appointed specifically to promote competitiveness and to gain a march on each other and on their purchasers. This is not fertile territory for the rebirth of a collective NHS and, although many new chairs and non-executive directors have been appointed to Trust Boards in the last few months, the executives remain the same individuals who were confronting their partners in the last contracting round.

Local authorities are also seen as key partners in delivering the new health agenda and in ensuring public accountability through their involvement in local health decision-making. There is no line management between central and local government and no existing duty on local authorities to take any interest in health matters. The strategy requires that this be changed and a statutory duty will be placed on local authorities to support the health agenda. It also appears that health authorities will be held to account for the performance of local authorities in their support role.

Direction, vision or detail?

The production of a comprehensive policy document, like this White Paper, naturally poses as many questions as it answers. The absence of detail in many of the proposals helps to avoid opposition at this early stage. As far as the principles go, there is unlikely to be systematic opposition as the proposals do offer a relatively painless way out of the stifling bureaucracy and increasing pointlessness of the NHS internal market. While Ministers profess to allow local solutions to emerge, that is not the style of the civil service. At least 62 working groups have been set up by the Department of Health to provide guidance on the issues raised in the White Paper; the fact that such guidance is not sought by the NHS does not affect this behaviour. At present, there is so much energy in NHS management to take forward the agenda described in the following pages that it is unlikely that the guidance will be in time; a case of guidance expected rather than guidance awaited.

In this book, I describe the main changes proposed in the White

Paper, the impact these changes will have on the working lives of health service staff, the underlying themes in policy which are driving the changes and the potential fulfilment of these policies for health and health care.

Part 2

The facts, the proposals, the reasons

The Foreword

Tony Blair's initial message sets the scene, placing the 'New NHS' in the context of its own history and, especially, the Labour Party's role in its creation. Apart from self-praise for the achievements so far in this Parliament (extra funding for the NHS, renewed private finance initiatives for hospitals and an investment focus on breast cancer and paediatric intensive care – rather cheekily described as 'children's services'), Blair introduces the new language of the NHS; replacing the internal market with integrated care, saving £1 billion of red tape, combining efficiency and quality with a belief in fairness and partnership – the language of the successful election campaign. The buzz word is modernization, characterized best by the desire to use electronic communications as effectively as in other industries such as banking. The promise of extra funding comes with a trade off; a responsibility within the service to change, to provide better care when it is needed and care of a uniformly high standard.

Modernization reflecting the expectations of our community requires a concerted effort at all levels. Modern Britain does not expect to wait for service, does expect full disclosure of detailed and relevant information and demands a style of service which puts the customer/user first. This is not yet the culture of the health care industry but we must assume that it will increasingly become so. The utterly negative images of older aspects of the NHS estate also need attention, although they are not addressed at all in this White Paper.

1

A modern and dependable NHS: there when you need it

Speed and efficiency

This is not a summary, more of a scene setting. Speed is the key issue and the analysis of weaknesses and solutions focuses on rapidity of response as the panacea. The problems of the NHS are described in terms of delays in treatment, variable quality and too much administration. There is a formal rejection of the widely held view that taxes (or charges) must rise or rationing must be introduced. Much is made of the variations in practice and variable efficiency and it is concluded that greater efficiency will deliver the resources required to enhance quality. It is implied that all variations can be abolished and that all providers can attain the standards of the best. Variations, however, are of two types: systematic variation which is due to controllable behaviour; and random variation which is due to chance. The former can be addressed by management action but random variation will always persist. The Government shows no sign of understanding this distinction.

The health of the people

The public health context is emphasized from the outset with a commitment to improve health and reduce inequalities in health, and the role of the Green Paper – *Our Healthier Nation* – is trailed. The Government gives itself 10 years to renew and improve the NHS, realistic in terms of the challenges and possibly in terms of electoral politics. The basic principle of local doctors and nurses having the best understanding of patients' needs is promoted but is extended, without evidence, to the task given to them in shaping local (specialist) services. This extrapolation of the principle is rejected by many consultants who have spent the last seven years defending their services against very mixed views and very variable knowledge of primary care commissioners. Indeed, there is no reason why generalists should be in any position to judge the value of specialists. Perhaps it is considered that they are better than anyone else and certainly better balanced in their views than the specialists themselves. There are consistent references to community nurses, partly to dilute the power of doctors, partly for populist reasons and least, perhaps, for their distinctive contribution.

Realizing the benefits of technology

The Government commits itself to achieving a goal which has eluded all its predecessors, namely the harnessing of information (communications) technology to the benefit of operational health services. Three symbolic examples of location are given to demonstrate the characteristics of a modernized NHS: at home, in the community and in hospital. Key elements of the new service will include a 24-hour telephone advice line staffed by nurses and giving health and health care advice to help people care for themselves at home (three pilot projects in Milton Keynes, Newcastle and Northumberland, and around Preston started operation in March 1998, universal coverage by 2000); by connecting all GP surgeries to the NHSnet, the results of investigations will be available faster and outpatient appointments can be booked direct (demonstration sites in each region by end of 1998, test results in all computerized practices by end of 1999 and in all practices by 2002); the symbol for hospitals will be guaranteed access to specialist assessment within two weeks for anyone with suspected cancer (breast cancer by 1999, all cancers one year later).

There will be those in the NHS who regard these targets as unachievable and others who consider them of subsidiary importance in the context of the problems facing the NHS. For example, no need has been demonstrated for a telephone advice line and no quantification of the impact exists. Banking has demonstrated the value of such a service to their business, but the NHS is a different sort of business. However, the real problem is that such proposals are startlingly unambitious for a truly modern health service. In most leading-edge health and health care systems for example, a two-day, rather than two-week, wait for investigation of possible cancer would be acceptable, yet there will be managers and clinicians who suggest that giving a two-week commitment will distort other priorities.

Waiting times again

In addition to these specific benefits, the Government repeats its commitment to reduce waiting lists by 100 000 (approximately 9%) during the life of this Parliament, a relaxation from the manifesto which promised this reduction within a year. This change is in recognition of the short-term pressures facing the NHS and postpones, but does not cancel, the commitment to reduce waiting times. After this initial relaxation of waiting lists, the Government is now pushing forward with targets for the reduction in numbers waiting as well as waiting times by the year 2002, i.e. the end of its five-year term. It has already been warned that, without extra resources, a 10% increase in efficiency will be required each year to achieve this goal. The Government's response includes additional funds (£500 million in 1998/99 on account) as well as threats to the livelihood of managers.

The funding is sufficient if we use it well

This chapter continues with an interesting analysis of the big picture for tax-funded health care. It rejects the notion that the challenges of balancing need, demand and affordability are too great to meet head on and promotes a rationalist view of a safe and successful future for the NHS. Specifically, it acknowledges that the demand side is rising through public expectation, medical techno-logical advances and demography (the ageing population). It makes the fascinating and probably true observations that the pressures on the NHS have always been exaggerated, the fact that 70% of the demographic pressures to confront the NHS in the 20 years from 1988 have already been accommodated and, more controversially, that technology and public health action will take the pressure off health care. This last point is almost certainly misguided.

The case for technology is based on several misconceptions. These include the idea that less invasive interventions are necessa-rily cheaper, that angioplasty (incorrectly described as 'heart catheters') will replace coronary artery bypass grafts, that day surgery replaces expensive inpatient care (partly true) and that successful public health action reduces the burden on health care services. In practice, while there is some truth in all but the last of these, the general trend is for new technologies to add to the scope and range of care options and not to substitute for existing ones. This is particularly so for minimally invasive surgery, angioplasty and day surgery, all of whose development has fuelled large increases in activity and overall increases in costs. The assumption that better public health will reduce the burden on the NHS is completely wrong. Effective public health postpones disease and death until old age when the burden of disease falls greater on health services due to the combined dependency of disease and the frailty of old age. A long-lived population experiences fewer early deaths but higher levels of chronic disability; this is the factor which converts ageing into care costs.

Keep the bureaucracy at bay

The case for rationing is rejected in favour of making better use of existing resources, especially through the diversion of management costs into frontline services. The magical figure of £1 billion is declared as a reduction in management costs over the lifetime of the current Parliament. This is already largely delivered – £500 million from the £100 million reduction declared in 1997/98 (× 5) and £320 million from the £80 million announced for 1998/99 (× 4). By the end of the Parliament, assuming that the remaining £180 million is released from 1999/2000 onwards, the annual saving on management costs compared with 1996/97 (the last full year of the last Government) will be £240 million, equivalent to 0.7% of NHS costs in England. There is also a firm lead on harnessing new developments rather than merely reacting to them. The systematic approach developed by the research and development strategy to testing and evaluating new technologies has to be translated into a systematic approach to basing clinical and managerial decisions on reliable evidence. The use of systematic cost-effectiveness evidence is also promoted, a signal that the rationing debate is not yet dead, merely relabelled. If only systematic cost-effectiveness evidence were widely available.

Power with responsibility for clinicians

A key innovation is the alignment of clinical and financial responsibility, effectively among groups of general practitioners. Professionals who make prescribing and referring decisions must now make these decisions in the best interests of their patients knowing that they have a single integrated budget to cover the costs. A framework of national service standards will ensure that strategies are consistent, but it is not clear how the much-vaunted fairness and consistency can be achieved with further delegation of decision-making.

The NHS is cheap

An unexpected claim is made in the penultimate paragraph, namely that the national economy depends on the NHS. This is not a repeat of the naiveté of the Beveridge proposals which anticipated that more health care would create a healthier and more efficient and productive workforce; it is a recognition that the low costs and efficiency of the NHS compared with other national health systems relieves the nation's industry of a major tax and/or cost burden.

2

A new start: what counts is what works

The third way

The Government rejects a return to the pre-reform structure, more because of the precedent it would set for other sectors than for its impact on the NHS. It also, of course, rejects the status quo and describes its proposals as *the third way*, implying a difference rather than a combination. The 'third way' terminology is appearing with increasing frequency in cabinet statements; it appears to seek a middle way between the social exclusion which results from unfettered capitalism and the stifling of energy which accompanies statism. It is an attempt to emulate the American Democratic Party, a one nation, socially conscious party which still upholds, with passion, the American dream. For the NHS context, this is the difference between the 'divisive internal market system (of the Tories)' and the 'command and control systems of the '70s (under both parties)'. Unfairness and bureaucracy are seen as the enemies and collaboration as the basic element of success. Six key principles are described (*see* Box 4) which underlie the changes proposed. These principles appear later under various guises including the performance framework.

> ## Box 4   Six key principles for *The New NHS*
>
> - A genuinely national service; fair access to consistently high-quality, prompt and accessible services
>
> - The delivery of health care against new national standards to be a matter of local responsibility
>
> - The needs of the patient will be put at the centre of the care process; the NHS will work in partnership with local authorities
>
> - Drive efficiency through a more rigorous approach to performance and by cutting bureaucracy
>
> - Shift the focus on to quality of care so that excellence is guaranteed and quality becomes the driving force
>
> - Rebuild public confidence in the NHS, accountable to patients, open to the public and shaped by their views

Among the 'not broken so won't be fixed' elements of the service it inherited, the Government will retain the separation between the planning of hospital care and its provision, the central role of primary care and the devolved responsibilities of trusts. The so-called purchaser/provider split is now confined to secondary care and is relabelled 'planning'. General practitioners are retained in pole position, against the core political philosophy, because it is impossible to control anything if they are outside the structure. The Government has been shrewd in amending its traditional stance on GPs and retaining them as key players, but I am less sure that they have judged the uncertain mood among GPs as keenly as they might. In particular, there is a need for visible and positive incentives for GPs to retain the enthusiasm they showed for fundholding in the face of vigorous opposition in 1991. Retaining trust freedoms for operational services merely recognizes the turmoil that any other strategy would entail and continues to locate some of the more serious service failures at some distance from the Government itself. It is often useful to have someone else to blame! In contrast, the proposals purport to end the fragmentation, unfairness, distortion, inefficiency, bureaucracy, instability and secrecy of the internal market.

Fragmentation

Here we are introduced to the idea that there are 4000 organizations in the NHS, comprising 100 health authorities, 400 trusts and
3500 GP fundholders. Much is made later of the reduction in the
number of NHS organizations but most would question whether
fundholding practices rate as organizations alongside either
existing health authorities and trusts or prospective primary care
groups. Notwithstanding the play on numbers, the introduction of
a local joint planning process, leading to the production of a jointly
agreed Health Improvement Programme is a clear signal to all
agencies that collectivism is back and, with the added involvement
of social care, with a vengeance.

Unfairness

It is implied that competition and unfairness are inevitable com-
panions and that the competitive values upset the sensitivities of
professional staff. While this is undoubtedly true up to a point, it
was the natural competitiveness of staff which drove the reforms of
the previous Government. Admittedly, some of this competitiveness, both of organizations and of individuals, was conceived in an
atmosphere of survival of the fittest and the competitive behaviour
which followed was clearly defensive in intent. However, repairing
the splits in professions created by optional structures, especially
fundholding, has been generally welcomed, suggesting a discom-
fort in the professions with competitiveness. Needs-based treatment
and professional co-operation are the new rules and influence is
guaranteed for community nurses, often the least consulted con-
stituency, and specialist clinicians, previously overconsulted prior
to the internal market.

Distortion

This may be regarded as overuse of the whip, describing the
natural behaviour of the marketplace in another way. Here it is the

commercial ownership of information and intellectual property which comes under the cosh. The answer will be the systematic sharing of best practice, and variable performance standards will be addressed by a new national performance framework covering the six key principles.

Inefficiency

This is an immensely popular and justified assault on the Purchaser Efficiency Index, arguably the most absurd performance monitoring vehicle yet invented in the UK. It measured change in the purchasing of health care at the margin and took it to describe performance at the core. It encouraged perverse activity and constituted a disincentive to effective care. For example, the desired reduction in unnecessary diagnostic Ds&Cs was complicated by the fact that they are usually performed as day cases, regarded as a universally good thing. Indeed, all activity was regarded as good, however pointless it may have been clinically. The separation of different parts of the NHS budget, long seen as a protection for patients, also comes in for criticism. The integration of budgets is a central element of the financial changes but may prove to be an Achilles heel if, for example, prescribing costs rise steeply – as has happened before – and impact on the funding of hospital services. We are promised better measures of real efficiency; the absence of detail or even ideas exposes the challenge in fulfilling the promise.

Bureaucracy

The implementation of the previous Government's reforms increased management costs by 1% of total NHS revenue. Recent cuts in management costs at all levels have already released more than this since 1993 but some of these reductions are masked by redefinitions. With such a busy management agenda, and with universal organizational change, further steep reductions in management seriously threaten the ability of the NHS to manage at all. The reduction of £1 billion during the lifetime of the Parliament is, as already indicated, a neat trick with numbers; statistically correct but of limited impact. As a manager, I would have to say that it could have been worse.

Instability

This is really about replacing contracts with agreements and substituting long-term arrangements for annual and cost-per-case contracts. In most places, the change will be modest because major shifts in services have been rare and most contracts are simply cost and activity rationalizations. It is the culture which will change rather than the currency. The inclusiveness of the Health Improvement Programme (medium-term plans agreed by all local agencies) and the unification of commissioning at primary care group and health authority level reduce the scale and frequency of change. There is little in the White Paper about the role of the private sector, but up to £100 million annually of fundholder expenditure on private providers could be restored to the NHS family over time.

Secrecy

An interesting departure into the original language of *Working for Patients*, which also used the term 'self-governing' to describe NHS trusts, introduces this conversion from commercialism to collectivism. Trust Boards are now required to meet in public, a new challenge for many members and one likely to result in much hard work for PR rescue merchants. We are also introduced to the publication of trust performance data, the real means of accountability, and the consequent naming and shaming which will inevitably result. Two other nuances are apparent: the greater openness at local level seeks to compensate for the continuation of central control of the NHS and the democratic deficit which so motivated Labour while in opposition; and a promise of additional funding each year but on condition that it delivers major gains in quality and efficiency. No change in policy there then.

3

Driving change in the NHS: quality and efficiency hand in hand

Restructure and change the paradigm

The new NHS structures and their roles are introduced together with the features of the new performance and quality standards. Quality is described in broad terms: doing the right things, at the right time, for the right people and doing them right first time – alternatively interpreted as effective, timely, appropriate and efficient. The process is important as well as the outcome.

Once again the internal market is portrayed as the criminal, distracting NHS staff from their main purpose. There is concern at serious lapses of quality which have harmed patients and dented public confidence. This is a reference to several failures of screening programmes for breast and cervical cancer and to errors in pathology and radiotherapy services. The experience of these, and the absence of any action against the professional culprits, is what lies behind the new statutory responsibility for quality and the accountability of trust chief executives. There is no mention of the powers which chief executives can exercise internally to deal with failing professionals; this is presumably too sensitive at this stage but is a necessary addition. If poor performance is to be eliminated, it must be made easier to dismiss incompetent doctors.

Quality

The example of the Calman–Hine report on the commissioning of cancer services, a unique exercise in central planning during the previous Government, is used to promote the advantages of the proposed evidence-based National Service Frameworks. As with the cancer strategy, the goal will be consistency of access to uniformly high-quality care.

A National Institute for Clinical Excellence will provide the long-awaited link between the NHS Research and Development strategy and the operational NHS. The Institute will draw up evidence-based guidelines for clinical services and disseminate them throughout the NHS; neither function is now performed.

At local level, the responsibility for raising the quality of services will fall to GPs and community nurses working together in primary care groups, service agreements between all NHS bodies encompassing national standards and a new system of clinical governance in all providers which is tantalizingly undefined. Of these, it is the clinical governance initiative which holds the key, together with the reserve powers retained by the Government to intervene. Such intervention will be triggered by reports from a new Commission for Health Improvement which will act as an inspectorial body for poorly performing providers.

Efficiency

Variations in efficiency are as unfair to patients as variations in quality, as inefficiency deprives patients of access to services. Five approaches are adopted to secure improvements in efficiency (*see* Box 5). The integration of budgets and the alignment of clinical and financial responsibility are acts of faith and I am not aware of any reason to assume that they will lead to greater efficiency – more likely that they will increase the risk to primary care group solvency. The reductions in management costs have largely been achieved already and the service is at risk of becoming undermanaged. The real crunch for providers is the proposed publication of reference costs and their imposition as standards to beat by trusts whose performance will be known and therefore published, though not necessarily by the Government – another example of naming and shaming. This is how costs will be reduced and resources released, or so the strategy assumes. The incentives and sanctions are less important for their ultimate value and more so for the impact they will have on the willingness of GPs to engage actively in primary care groups, an engagement which is in the balance at this stage.

Box 5   Ensuring efficiency in *The New NHS*

- Aligning clinical and financial responsibility and devolving responsibility for a single unified budget to primary care groups; this will cover most services and will offer incentives at group and practice level

- Management costs will be capped in health authorities and primary care groups and reduced in trusts

- The Government will publish reference costs for individual treatments and will require trusts to make known, and to benchmark, their own costs

- There will be cash incentives to improve performance and efficiency for health authorities, trusts and primary care groups

- Sanctions can be imposed on poor performers including withdrawal of freedoms (from primary care groups) and the right to move services between providers is retained. Direct intervention by the NHS Executive is also possible

Measurement

The new performance framework, measuring health improvement, fairer access to services, quality and outcomes, the views of patients and real efficiency, is introduced briefly on the principle of what gets measured gets done. In the past, the wrong things were measured and management was perverse, i.e. it addressed the measured elements rather than the important things, and the wrong measures produced the wrong results. This is fair comment but it is not easy to monitor performance against things we have never measured and data we do not collect. The Government appears willing to invest in information technology to overcome this problem and is determined to successfully apply technological solutions to the age-old challenge of health data which are timely, relevant and of high quality. However, the examples given (*see* Box 6) have the appearance of a textbook rather than a strategy which is realizable.

Box 6 Information technology for quality and efficiency

- Making patients' records electronically available

- Using the NHSnet and the Internet to deliver test results quickly, online booking of appointments and up-to-date advice

- Prompt financial and performance information

- Using the Internet and digital TV to provide knowledge on health, illness and treatment for the public

- Introducing telemedicine to disseminate specialist skills to all parts of the country

---

Roles and responsibilities

The roles of the main structures of the new NHS are outlined, with more detailed analysis in subsequent chapters. The health authorities will be the planning agencies, primary care groups are the focus of integrated care, trusts will be specialist providers and the Department of Health will integrate health and social care policy and will try to control the professions.

4

Health authorities: leading and shaping

In charge

Health authorities will be the strategic leaders of the local NHS and their stronger role will overcome the fragmentation of previous structures and especially the internal market. This is a criticism of the freedoms given to both trusts and fundholders in the previous reforms. Health authority functions are summarized in Box 7.

> ### Box 7   The functions of the new health authorities
>
> - Assessing the health needs of the local population
>
> - Drawing up a Health Improvement Programme to meet those needs, in partnership with local interests
>
> - Deciding the range and location of health care services for the authority's residents
>
> - Setting local targets and standards to drive quality and efficiency and ensuring their delivery

- Supporting the development of primary care groups
- Allocating resources to primary care groups
- Holding primary care groups to account

Health first

Public health policy is the lead-off point, enshrined in a new statutory duty to improve the health of populations. Health authorities will work with local authorities and others to identify local action, and public health action will include communicable disease control, health needs assessment, monitoring health outcomes and evaluating the health impact of local plans and developments. There is nothing new in any of this but health authorities have always had to do other things on which their performance was judged – public health performance has not been important hitherto until things go wrong. The Director of Public Health annual report will be the starting point for the Health Improvement Programme (HIP). To achieve this, the reports and the public health function will both have to improve greatly.

The HIP will be the local health and health care strategy and will detail how national targets are to be met. Health authorities will lead the other NHS and local authority organizations and the independent contractor professions in developing the HIP. Local authorities and NHS bodies will have a statutory responsibility of partnership. The HIP will cover the health needs of the population, the health care requirements to meet those needs and the range, location and investment in health services which are required. The programme will be a three-year rolling plan with annual updates. As they are responsible for the delivery of the NHS components of the plan, health authorities will have reserve powers over trust spending decisions, including capital plans and new consultant posts. The health authorities are also given responsibility for co-ordinating workforce education plans and, of more urgency, co-ordinating information and information technology plans across the whole of the NHS in their area. (This includes the development of primary care computing and managing 'the year 2000 problem' with computer chips. Health authorities do not have the skills to do this but then nor does anyone else in the NHS.) Co-operation with local authorities is seen as a problem and in future health authorities and social services will have to produce joint investment plans for continuing health and community care needs. Indeed, it is certainly possible that this framework could replace existing social services responsibility for the production of children's services plans and the annual community care plan. Pooled budgets and other stimuli to close working are envisaged.

Devolving commissioning but staying in control

Health authorities will devolve responsibility for commissioning of services to primary care groups as soon as possible. This harnesses the strategic view of health authorities and the innovative energies of primary care. However, health authorities will probably still be responsible for commissioning highly specialized tertiary services, under collaborative arrangements to be determined by NHS Executive Regional Offices, on which a consultation paper was published in April 1998.

The national targets set out in *Our Healthier Nation* will form the basis of HIPs to improve health, and primary care groups will have to commission services accordingly. Primary care groups and trusts will be held to account for delivering their elements of the programme and any disputes will be resolved by health authorities – this gives them a responsibility previously held by regional health authorities.

Accountable to the people

In addition to these management functions, health authorities will be expected to involve local people more effectively to build a new public confidence in the NHS. Using the simple maxim of the NHS being responsive and accountable, health authorities will involve the public in developing the HIP, ensure that primary care groups involve the public, publish their strategies, and progress and participate in the new user and patient survey. It is, in my view, unlikely that any of these actions will increase public confidence; that will only come from more tangible investment in the NHS, rising standards of service and fewer complaints of cuts and crises from staff.

The Government will enable these actions to be realized (*see* Box 8) and this may lead to fundamental changes in the existing framework of NHS organizations. For example, aligning trust and primary care group accountabilities with the HIP may lead to changes in authority boundaries. This will distort co-terminosity between NHS and local authorities, though this may matter less if social care responsibilities are increasingly integrated at primary care group level. The provision for local authority chief executives to participate in health authority meetings has aroused mixed feelings, especially among elected members of local authorities. The Government does not have the same management relationship with local authorities as it has with the NHS, nor does it seem to be particularly interested in the maintenance of long-standing local democratic structures, preferring to prepare for the devolution of government services to regional assemblies in its second term. Also, the role of chief executives in local authorities is less pre-eminent than in health authorities, while the role of the council leader is infinitely more so than that of NHS trust and health authority chairs. This proposal may well be rethought during future consultation although the advantages of working through officers are the avoidance of petty politics, accusations of bias and contamination with growing local sleaze.

Box 8 Making it happen

- Health authorities will have statutory responsibilities for improving the health of the population, and for working in partnership with other organizations

- NHS trusts and primary care groups will be responsible for working within the Health Improvement Programme and their responsibilities will be aligned within the health authority role

- Local authority chief executives will participate in meetings of health authorities; the experience of Health Action Zones will guide further strengthening of health and local authority partnership arrangements

- Health authority administrative functions will be shared and streamlined, to release time, effort and resources (for the new role); fewer authorities covering larger areas will emerge as a result

Radical centralization for GP administration

Of more profound significance to health authorities in the medium term is the so-called streamlining of their administrative functions. This is a euphemism for the centralization of the administration of independent contractors, a role which currently occupies about one third of their staff. Ultimately, within 10 years, there could be a single national agency for contractor support administration; in the interim, regional or sub-regional agencies will be established within two or three years with rationalization into one or two agencies per region. As we shall see, the number of independent contractors may well be declining sharply by this time.

5

Primary care groups: going with the grain

Still a primary care-led NHS?

The Government does a fair job of declaring its support for broadly based primary care services. Their description covers the full range of professions and the great scope for the development of their role in the future. While recognizing the importance of general practice, it is clear that the development of primary and community care lies largely in other areas of the service. While the independent contractor status of GPs is not directly affected by the proposals, over time alternatives will grow in number and attractiveness.

Learning from experience: primary care groups

The Government's proposals are allegedly based on the success of recent collective approaches to primary care-led commissioning, such as total purchasing pilots and multifunds, despite the absence of any completed evaluation of them. The merits of empowering primary care are accepted without reservation as is the rejection of a competitive market. Primary care groups will be the manifestation of the new arrangement and unlike existing schemes, they will be mandatory and universal, with a uniform structure and progressive responsibilities. Their functions, structure and requirements are summarized in Boxes 9, 10 and 11.

Box 9   The main functions of primary care groups

- Contribute to the health authority's Health Improvement Programme on health and health care, reflecting the perspective of the local community and the experience of patients

- Promote the health of the local population, in partnership with other agencies

- Commission health services from relevant NHS trusts, within the framework of the Health Improvement Programme

- Monitor performance against the service agreements they have with NHS trusts

- Develop primary care by joint working across practices; sharing skills; providing a forum for professional development, audit and peer review; developing the new approach to clinical governance

- Integrate primary and community health services and work more closely with social services on planning and delivery

---

Box 10   Options for the scope and responsibilities of primary care groups

- **TIER 1** Advise and support the health authority in commissioning care for its population

- **TIER 2** Take devolved responsibility for managing the budget for health care in their area, formally as part of the health authority

- **TIER 3**   Become established as freestanding bodies accountable to the health authority for commissioning care

- **TIER 4**   As Tier 3 but with added responsibility for the provision of community health services for their population (primary care trusts)

Box 11   Common core requirements for primary care groups

- Representative of all the general practices in the group

- A governing body which includes community nursing and social services as well as GPs drawn from the area

- Take account of social services boundaries as well as health authority areas to help promote integration in service planning and provision

- Abide by the local Health Improvement Programme

- Clear arrangements for public involvement including open meetings

- Efficient and effective arrangements for management and financial accountability

---

We can draw a number of inferences from the presentation of these characteristics. First, it is clear that primary care groups will be more like health authorities than any of the various forms of primary care commissioning now operating. In particular, primary care trusts will be vertically integrated organizations with responsibility for both the provision and the commissioning of health services. Second, the structural inclusion of community nursing and social care is both a logical boost to the integration of care and a systematic attempt to dilute the power and influence of doctors in these groups. Third, while there are four options for the development and scope of responsibilities of the groups, and groups will declare their own position on the scale at the outset, there is only one direction to travel (towards Tier 4) and the overall strategy requires primary care groups to reach Tier 3 quickly, say by 2001 at the latest. This is to enable health authorities to slim down and focus on their new role, relieved of the responsibility for commissioning services. Fourth, the potential creation of primary care trusts, the first of which might be set up as early as 1999 – subject to legislation – has profound implications for existing NHS trusts. As primary care trusts will manage community health services and community hospitals, these will have to be removed from existing trusts. Furthermore, a late decision by the NHS Executive to exclude mental health and learning disability services from primary care groups, and the statement preferring specialist mental health trusts for these services, fundamentally changes NHS trust configuration in many places. We face a service model in no more than four years where all primary and community services may be managed by primary care trusts (including community hospitals), all mental health services and learning disability services will be in specialist NHS trusts and the general and specialist hospital services will be all that remains for other NHS trusts. Radical reconfiguration of NHS trusts is now under way to establish these frameworks with general support from Labour MPs and from Ministers. I understand that there are second thoughts about the independence of primary care trusts and especially their role as employers of community staff. It is being considered safer for health authorities to be the employers of convenience for these staff until primary care trusts have proved themselves.

A conundrum over mental health

There has been some discord in the Department of Health over the exclusion of mental health and learning disability services from primary care groups. The main concern of the proposers of these exclusions was the need to protect mental health services for political reasons, service failures being a particularly sensitive issue for Ministers. However, the transfer of community services to primary care groups will leave mental health services in limbo – their combination with acute general hospitals being regarded as unacceptable. Subsequent softening of the line suggests that once the new specialist trust arrangements are secure, community-based services for these groups may transfer to primary care groups and trusts.

Local and accountable

These primary care arrangements will be accountable to health authorities just as total purchasing pilots and multifunds are. They will cover populations of approximately 100 000 with a lower limit of about 50 000 and an, as yet, undeclared upper limit a little above 150 000. Further guidance has been issued on the rules of configuration and it is possible that groups can cross health authority boundaries and individual practices may be able to choose which group, and therefore which health authority, they are part of. Such changes are likely to be exceptional. Despite the inevitable guidance, it is understood that locally agreed proposals are likely to be accepted. These moves may well affect the subsequent redrawing of health authority boundaries. The budgets available to these primary care groups will be substantial (*see* Box 12) and, for the first time, bring together all the costs of treating patients in the NHS. It is presumed that the integration of these budgets with financial and clinical responsibility will improve the quality of decision-making. This may be true but only the prescribing budgets will be practice-based initially. Later, indicative budgets will be extended for all aspects of NHS expenditure to practices but this will be to sharpen accountability, not to delegate control. All decisions by primary care groups will be group-based; collectivism is back, individuality is relegated. However, groups may develop practice-based incentives in the future. There are basic flaws in these assumptions; if peer pressure is to be brought to bear on outlying practices (in terms of clinical behaviour and costs), then practice-level data will be required. However, the abandonment of practice-level data collection is a basic component of the abolition of fundholding and the move towards collective approaches to primary care-based commissioning. It is also necessary to stop collecting data in both commissioners and providers if the transaction costs of the internal market are to be slashed. At some point, the obsession with reducing management costs will abate and the need to secure control over expenditure will achieve precedence; perhaps practice-level data have not seen their armageddon just yet.

Box 12   Unified primary care group budgets

- The budget for the commissioning of all hospital and community health services

- The budget for the costs of drugs prescribed in primary care by doctors and nurses (there is an area of uncertainty here about the drugs prescribed by dentists)

- The cash-limited budget for general medical services infrastructure, used to reimburse practices for a proportion (usually 70%) of the cost of their practice staff and to meet part or all of the cost of practice premises and computers

- The total budget for the average primary care group will be over £50 million at 1998/99 value

Managing the drug budget

The undoubted, if relative, success of the fundholding scheme in controlling the rise in expenditure of pharmaceuticals lies behind the integration of prescribing budgets with the commissioning funds for hospital and community health services. It also creates the Treasury's dream of at last being able to stop worrying about the rising drug bill; that pleasure now belongs to primary care groups as any rise in drug costs must be compensated for by a reduction in hospital costs. At approximately 10% of the total NHS cost, drugs are a major but not overwhelming component of NHS costs and pressures. In recent years, the proportion has started to rise and, as more expensive and effective drugs make their way on to the market, drugs will continue to increase as a share of total NHS expenditure. There is nothing wrong with this growth so long as the new drugs provide clinical value. Also, the fraught interface between hospital prescribing and community prescribing can now be relaxed, but the preferential prices at which drugs are sold to hospitals could now be under threat. There is also clear evidence that dispensing practices are disincentivized from delivering efficient prescribing, an issue which requires complex action. The Government will also find itself grappling with the tense relationship that its predecessors enjoyed with the pharmaceutical industry, especially in terms of the NHS drug pricing regime. It has already indicated that the recovery of research and development costs through drug prices has such an impact on the total cost that the volume of R&D whose costs are recovered in this way might usefully be reviewed (downwards).

Tough times for fundholding staff

Because the whole primary care group concept is based on collective approaches, little of the existing administration associated with practice level involvement in fundholding will be required. The management costs should therefore be substantially reduced. Health authorities will have a management cost envelope which will cover their own costs and those of the primary care groups. This will be set at a level below that which most currently have for health authority and fundholding management costs. However, the 10% cut in the fundholder management allowance for 1998/99 narrows the gap, and operating within the cost envelope should not be difficult if duplication of data collection is avoided. However, NHS trusts must be able to demonstrate that they can deliver high-quality data which have the confidence of general practitioners; this has not generally been the case with fundholders. The White Paper includes a figure of £3 per head of population to support the running costs of primary care groups. In fact this is just an averaging of the surviving fundholder management allowance (after incremental cuts) shared equally across the country. Primary care groups will also have a share of the health authority's commissioning costs to work with and, in Tier 4, a share of the management costs of community health services. For a population of 100 000, a primary care trust may well have management cost allowances of well over £500 000.

Primary care trusts: into the (un)known

Further guidance is expected on the criteria and board structure for primary care trusts. It is clear, however, that they will remain accountable to health authorities, unlike NHS trusts, and will have to comply with corporate and clinical governance rules including the appointment of accountable officers, probably the chair or the chief executive. Such is the scale and scope of these responsibilities that they are likely to be fulfilled by professional managers and not by general practitioners. This is the clearest signal that primary care groups are not a development of fundholding but are a localization of health authorities with the integration of primary and community care within a single accountable body, possibly with social care to follow.

The management implications

The level of management which has become commonplace in fundholding practices and in operational services in community care is characteristic of middle management, craving certainty and hoarding information. The type of management required for Tier 3 commissioning primary care groups and, especially, Tier 4 commissioning and providing primary care trusts is very much higher. These more senior and capable managers thrive on paradox and on uncertainty; their turnover in posts is higher, they take more risks and their approach is more appropriate to the excitement which trust status introduces. These management skills are only available in NHS trusts and health authorities, and just possibly some of the most advanced total purchasing pilots, and this is where the top managers of primary care trusts will come from.

The other professions

There are brief references to the roles of health visitors in commissioning and the one and only mention of the other contractor professions (dentistry, pharmacy and optometry) with no real idea of how they fit in – because they don't. The flexibility of the *NHS (Primary Care) Act 1997* is retained as the vehicle for developing primary and community services. This, together with the potential ability for primary care trusts to renegotiate the GMS contract locally, signals the possible end for independent contractor status in some areas. The persistent references to the retention of this status throughout the White Paper suggests that there is fire behind the smoke.

Herding cats

Quality and effectiveness also get a shove in the form of promised indicators to assess the effectiveness of primary care at national and health authority level. Furthermore, each primary care group will have to develop and promote clinical governance and professional development, with senior professional leadership at both group and practice level. This suggests a fairly low level of understanding, by the authors, of the dynamics of general practice. The evidence from new arrangements for providing GMS cover out of hours suggests that GPs can work together when it is in their own interests to do so. Peer review, however, is not part of the culture.

Not so fast and not so simple

Finally, there is a flash of recognition that undoing the eight years of fundholding in a period of 15 months from the publication of the White Paper may create some little local difficulty. For example, a high proportion of staff employed by practices under the fundholding scheme will be redundant and their skills may well not be required by the new groups. Such affected staff include not only managers associated with the fundholding scheme, but also clinical staff – especially nurses – whose skills are still required but who only became affordable because of the management allowance for fundholding. Who bears the cost of redundancy? Who handles appointments of staff to the primary care groups? Who compensates practices for severance costs? Should anyone compensate small businesses (although their involvement in fundholding in the first place was at the Government's request, they have been amply rewarded)? What do practices do with the space occupied by fundholding staff, often extensions paid for with savings from the fundholding scheme? What happens to the retained savings from the scheme (perhaps £200 million nationally)?

Many of these questions have been at least partly answered by HSC 1998 (065), the guidance on establishing primary care groups. Early departure from fundholding is hoped to release resources to cover interim costs; severance costs will be borne by the management allowance, the fund (including savings) or the health authority – in that order; the remaining savings will be made available to primary care groups. However, internal practice issues remain unresolved.

6

NHS trusts: partnership and performance

Just following orders

Trusts are seen as the victims of the market rather than its creators. They are now given the opportunity to make good by focusing on quality and efficiency (*see* Box 13). There is little new in this except clinical governance, still tantalizingly undefined, and the rules on openness already implemented.

Box 13   A new paradigm for NHS trusts

- NHS trusts will participate in strategy and planning by helping shape the Health Improvement Programme

- New standards for quality and efficiency, explicit in local agreements (between health authorities, primary care groups and NHS trusts) alongside new measures of efficiency

- Doctors, nurses and other senior professionals will be more closely involved in designing service agreements with commissioners, and in aligning NHS trust financial priorities with clinical priorities

- Clinical governance arrangements will be developed in all NHS trusts to guarantee an emphasis on quality

- NHS trusts will be able to share and invest efficiency gains to improve services consistent with the Health Improvement Programme

- Public confidence will be rebuilt through openness, improved governance and public commitment to the value and aims of the NHS

Remarriage is on the cards

While retaining their independence as corporate organizations, NHS trusts must now work in local partnerships and can only use NHS funds for the collective NHS agenda – the Health Improvement Programme. This is a fundamental change in culture for many trusts and not one which will necessarily come naturally. As elsewhere, there is a boost for nursing as an independent profession with a distinctive contribution to make. The main thrust, however, is on quality and the most detailed account yet of clinical governance (*see* Box 14).

Box 14 Characteristics of a quality organization exercising clinical governance

- Quality improvement, e.g. clinical audit, is in place and integrated with the quality programme for the whole organization

- Leadership skills are developed for each clinical team

- Evidence-based practice is in day-to-day use with infrastructure to support it

- There is systematic dissemination (inside and outside the organization) of evaluated good practice, ideas and innovations

- High-standard clinical risk reduction programmes are in place

- Adverse events are detected, openly investigated and the lessons learned are promptly applied

- Lessons for clinical practice, from complaints by patients, are systematically learned

- Poor clinical performance is recognized at an early stage and dealt with to prevent harm to patients

- Professional development programmes reflect the principles of clinical governance

- High-quality data are collected to monitor clinical care

Clinical quality first

Every NHS trust will have to embrace the concept of clinical governance so that quality is at the core of organizational and professional responsibilities. New legislation will give them a new duty for quality of care and chief executives will carry ultimate responsibility for assuring the quality of care. Appropriate local arrangements, such as a Board sub-committee led by a senior clinical professional, will be put in place to ensure the internal clinical governance of the organization. These arrangements, which strengthen existing professional self-regulation, will extend to engage professionals at ward and clinical level. Monthly reports on quality will be presented to NHS trust boards together with an annual report. This is all very open and up front; it is also a manifestation of this Government's favourite tool of control: naming, shaming and blaming. While there is a degree of moral superiority in the approach, it is hardly compatible with a statutory duty of partnership. Engaging professionals in their own public humiliation is not likely to be a popular strategy with the people who actually make up the NHS, the health professionals.

Sanctions galore

The performance of NHS trusts, the tools for which are covered in more detail elsewhere, is also hard-hitting. A new, broadly based performance framework, accountability through service agreements, accountable to the NHS Executive for statutory quality and financial performance – who wants to be a trust chief executive? Furthermore, for miscreants there is a new formal five-stage system for taking NHS trusts to the brink of destruction (*see* Box 15). In fact, the only new bit of this is the Commission for Health Improvement. It must be rather reassuring to NHS trusts that the removal of services comes at the fourth level and just before the removal of the trust itself!

Box 15   Investigation and intervention for failing NHS trusts

1 Health authorities call in the NHS Executive Regional Offices when an NHS trust is failing to deliver against the Health Improvement Programme

2 NHS Executive Regional Offices will investigate where there may be a failure to comply with statutory duties

3 The Commission for Health Improvement will be called in to investigate and report on problems

4 Primary care groups will be able to change their local service agreements where NHS trusts are failing to deliver

5 The Secretary of State can remove NHS trust boards

Lower management and procedure costs

Under the heading of efficiency, despite a lot of words, it is hard to find anything really encouraging for NHS trusts. In fact, it is difficult to find anything at all except cuts in costs. Procedure costs will be benchmarked and published, management costs will be reduced by abolishing the transactions of the internal market and extra-contractual referrals, and managers will be able to focus on managing not bureaucracy, but they won't be managing integrated hospital and community services, a service model which is now officially frowned upon.

Looking after staff

The Government wants to be seen as kinder to staff than its predecessor and there are a lot of positive words to this end. Various initiatives are described in Box 16. The biggest problem, however, is the chaos which local pay determination has imposed on pay structures. To convert from local pay to national pay would bring two seriously unwanted problems. First, average pay would rise leading to cuts in services; second, some staff would lose pay – after protection – leading to staff dissatisfaction. To avoid these risks, and because it doesn't know what to do, the Government treats this as a long-term issue and the topic of discussions.

Box 16   Involving staff in NHS trusts

- Moving towards national pay with meaningful local flexibility

- Action on issues which affect the quality of working lives of NHS staff

- Immediate priority to:
  - minimize accidents at work
  - avoid violence at work
  - address stress from work
  - recognize and deal with racism
  - flexible, family-friendly employment policies
  - reasonable standards of food and accommodation for on-call doctors
  - enable staff to speak out when necessary without victimization

- Involving staff in planning service developments and changes

- A taskforce on involving frontline staff in shaping new patterns of health care

- NHS trust boards will have to review regularly their success in involving staff

- Publication in NHS trust annual reports of their policy on staff involvement and the outcome of negotiations or initiatives

Greater involvement of staff, together with open meetings, more representative boards and the publication of information are all designed to help build public confidence in the structures and ethos of the NHS, confidence which was dented during the turbulent years around the previous reforms. No such turbulence is apparent yet but discord with staff over the phasing of their pay awards, further bed closures and a fight back against external regulation by the medical profession are all likely in the near future.

7

The national dimension: a one nation NHS

Tough at the top

While one can understand the presentational importance of starting with local structures and working up to the centre, this is not quite what has been offered. We are first offered a new strategic role for health authorities, then the new primary care groups which take on some old health authority functions, then NHS trusts with a new paradigm and limited emasculation; now for the Department of Health, pre-eminent as always.

Unified policies

The Department, we are told, will integrate policy on public health, social care and the NHS so that there is a clear national framework for similar local development – great. The NHS Executive will develop and implement policy for the NHS – fine. Management costs for the Department of Health and the NHS Executive will be subject to the same rigour as those of the NHS – good. As fewer and larger health authorities emerge, the role of NHS Executive Regional Offices will need to be kept under review – this means they will either be abolished, with health authorities becoming the regions, or they will be reduced in number to, say, two. Either way, the impact on the centre will be profound. The worst outcome could be that health authorities are absorbed into the NHS Executive, replacing the Regional Offices, which would again deprive the operational NHS of any strategic role, increase the role of the civil service and reduce the career options for senior staff in the NHS.

NICE, CHIMP and NSFs

There is a national drive for quality and clinical effectiveness too, bearing down on unjustifiable variations in the application of evidence of clinical- and cost-effectiveness (*see* Box 17). This is a very strong framework if it can be realized. The R&D strategy is already in place, although there has been a long dispute over which branch of the NHS Executive has responsibility for the dissemination of the results of research. The National Service Frameworks are to be based on the cancer services model which has proved to be a unifying force and has led to improvements in local services. The intention is to publish a further two National Service Frameworks each year: priorities for 1999 will be mental health and coronary heart disease. The two new bodies are best known for their populist acronyms (NICE and CHIMP); neither currently exists, although I understand that NICE (*see* Box 18) will be placed in the arena of the professional Royal Colleges.

The repeated references to cost-effectiveness may suggest that the Government is really serious about making choices of priorities on the basis of the value of the benefits for patients. Indeed, the absence of any reference to comprehensiveness in all the descriptions of the new NHS suggests that the Government may have privately acknowledged that some limitations of scope for tax-funded health care may well be necessary and it is putting in place the justification for the tough decisions which follow in the future.

Box 17 The national initiative on clinical- and cost-effectiveness

- The research and development programme will ensure the provision and dissemination of high-quality scientific evidence on the cost-effectiveness and quality of care

- A programme of new evidence-based National Service Frameworks will set out patterns and levels of service which should be provided for patients with certain conditions

- A new National Institute for Clinical Excellence (NICE) will promote clinical and cost-effectiveness by producing clinical guidelines and audits for dissemination throughout the NHS

- A new Commission for Health Improvement (CHIMP) will support and oversee the quality of clinical governance and of clinical services

- Work with the professions to strengthen existing systems of professional self-regulation

Box 18 The National Institute for Clinical Excellence

- New coherence and prominence to information about clinical- and cost-effectiveness

- It will produce and disseminate:
  - clinical guidelines based on relevant evidence of clinical- and cost-effectiveness
  - clinical audit methodologies and information on good practice in clinical audit

- Bring together work done by many professional organizations receiving Department of Health funding

- Work to a programme agreed with the Department of Health

- Funded from resources already committed to this work (actually overheads disinvested from Royal Colleges funding in 1997/98)

- Membership will be drawn from the health professions, the NHS, academics, health economists and patient interests

This is an important discipline and would take the boldness and intellectual status of the Government's approach into uncharted waters. CHIMP, on the other hand, is more like an inspectorate along the lines of OFSTED, though presumably on a much smaller scale. It appears, however, to have the same powers of naming and shaming as OFSTED and the Secretary of State for Health will have the same range of powers over failing health services as the Secretary of State for Education and Employment has over schools.

New powers for Regional Directors

There is no change in the accountability of health authorities and NHS trusts to regional offices of the NHS Executive, though the issues on which they are held to account will change as previously described. Informal arrangements whereby Regional Directors are involved in the appointment of chief executives of health authorities and NHS trusts are now formalized, an important symbol of the integration of the NHS and reduced independence for each of its quangos.

Protection for specialist regional services

NHS Executive Regional Offices are given a new function in providing the means to commission specialist hospital services. This is to ensure fair access to highly specialized services where one provider meets the needs of more than one health authority. There are already national commissioning arrangements in place for those services where one provider meets the needs of more than one region, such as high-security psychiatric hospitals, liver transplantation and complex cranio-facial surgery. The precise range of services to be covered by these new regional arrangements is not yet known and may be for local agreement (*see* p. 92). Some groups of health authorities are already working together to commission specialist regional services. They do so by building on commissioning expertise which they possess for their mainstream commissioning responsibilities. By 2001, health authorities will not be heavily engaged in commissioning so a different arrangement may be necessary. Specialized commissioning units may be set up in regional offices as third party agencies or in one health authority acting on behalf of several authorities. In the longer term, these specialist commissioning arrangements could be harmonized with the redrawing of health authority boundaries covering populations in excess of one million.

8

Measuring progress: better every year

A new performance framework

The accountability of any body is limited by what is measured; the new performance framework sets out to define what it is important to do well and therefore what should be measured. The White Paper is less precise on the detail but further information has since been published as a consultation paper.

The six dimensions of success

The new framework has six dimensions (*see* Box 19). This will provide a much more rounded measure of NHS performance, among the best of any public service, and much more relevant to what the public and the professions want. The difficulty is not with the intent or with the acceptance of the intent by the NHS, but with developing robust and reliable measures of the six dimensions. In the consultation paper published in January 1998, a suggested set of high-level indicators is outlined (*see* Box 20). It is intended that

the framework should be useful to, and used by, the general public
– to inform them about their local NHS and to inform decisions
about their own care; NHS agencies – to inform and improve
performance and to use in planning; and Ministers and the NHS
Executive – to drive improvements in performance of health authorities and to demonstrate public accountability for the use of NHS
resources.

**Box 19 Six dimensions of the new National Perfor-
mance Framework**

- Health improvement:
  - reflecting the overall aim of improving the general health of
    the population, influenced by many factors beyond the NHS,
    e.g. changes in premature death rates, reflecting social and
    economic factors

- Fair access:
  - the NHS contribution must offer fair access to health services
    in relation to need, irrespective of geography, class, ethnicity,
    age or sex, e.g. ensuring that black and minority ethnic
    groups are not disadvantaged in terms of access

- Effective delivery of appropriate health care:
  - care must be effective, appropriate and timely, and comply
    with agreed standards, e.g. increasing provision of treatments
    of proven benefit (such as hip replacement), provision of
    rehabilitation at the point when it can offer most benefit,
    sustained delivery of health and social care to those with long-
    term needs, reducing inappropriate treatments

- Efficiency:
  - how the NHS uses its resources to achieve value for money,
    e.g. length of stay in hospital, day surgery, unit costs, labour
    productivity, management costs, capital utilization

- Patient/carer experience:
  - measuring how patients and carers view the quality of the
    treatment and care they receive
  - a new national patient survey and a new NHS Charter

- Health outcomes of NHS care:
  - assess the direct contribution of NHS care to improvements in health, e.g. trends in infectious diseases for which immunization is available

---

Box 20   Proposed set of high-level performance indicators

Health improvement

- Deaths from all causes (for people aged 15–64)
- Deaths from all causes (for people aged 65–74)
- Cancer registrations – the summation of age and sex standardized rates for the following cancers:
  - stomach
  - small intestine, colon, rectum, rectosigmoid junction, anus
  - trachea, bronchus and lung
  - malignant melanoma
  - non-melanoma skin cancer
  - female breast
  - cervix uteri

Fair access

- Surgery rates – a composite indicator of elective surgery rates, consisting of age and sex standardized:
  - CABG and PTCA rates
  - hip replacement rates (for those over 65)
  - knee replacement rates (for those over 65)
  - cataract replacement rates
- Conceptions below age 16 – measuring access to family planning services
- People registered with a NHS dentist – % of population registered
- Early detection of cancer – a composite indicator, consisting of:
  - % of target population screened for breast cancer
  - % of target population screened for cervical cancer

- District nurse contacts – a composite indicator looking at access to community services, consisting of:
  - district nurse contacts for those aged 75 and over
  - district nurse contacts over 30 mins for those aged 75 and over
  - assisted district nurse contacts for those aged 75 and over

Effective delivery of appropriate health care

- Disease prevention and health promotion – a composite indicator consisting of:
  - % of target population vaccinated
  - % of all orchidopexies below age five

- Early detection of cancer – a composite indicator of breast and cervical cancer screening as above

- Inappropriately used surgery – a composite indicator consisting of age and sex standardized:
  - rates of Ds&Cs performed in women under 40
  - surgical intervention rates for glue ear

- Surgery rates – a composite indicator of elective surgery rates for CABG, PTCA, hip and knee replacement and cataract replacement as above

- Acute care management – a composite indicator consisting of age and sex standardized admission rates for:
  - severe ENT infection
  - kidney/urinary tract infection
  - heart failure

- Chronic care management – a composite indicator consisting of age and sex standardized admission rates for:
  - asthma
  - diabetes
  - epilepsy

- Mental health in primary care – a composite indicator consisting of:
  - volume of benzodiazepines
  - ratio of antidepressants to benzodiazepines prescribed

- Cost-effective prescribing – a composite measure consisting of:
  - cost/ASTRO-PU of combination products
  - cost/ASTRO-PU of modified release products
  - cost/ASTRO-PU of drugs of limited clinical value
  - cost/ASTRO-PU of inhaled corticosteroids
- Discharge from hospital – a composite indicator consisting of:
  - rate of discharge home within 56 days of emergency admission from home with a stroke
  - rate of discharge home within 56 days of admission with a fractured neck of femur

Efficiency

- Day case rate

- Length of stay in hospital (casemix adjusted)

- Unit cost (HCHS)

- Generic prescribing (%)

Patient/carer experience of the NHS

- Patients who wait more than two hours for emergency admission (admitted through A&E)

- Patients with operations cancelled for non-medical reasons on the day of, or after, admission

- Delayed discharge from hospital for people aged over 75 (per 1000 75-year-olds not in hospital)

- First outpatient appointments for which patient did not attend (%)

- Outpatients seen within 13 weeks of GP referral (%)

- Inpatients admitted within three months of a decision to admit (%)

Health outcomes of NHS care

- Conceptions below age 16

- Decayed, missing and filled teeth in five-year olds

- Avoidable diseases – a composite indicator of avoidable diseases and impairments, consisting of age and sex standardized:
  - notification rates for pertussis in children
  - notification rates for measles
  - episode rates for fracture of proximal femur (in those aged 65 and over)
  - notification rates for TB

- Adverse events/complications of treatment – a composite indicator consisting of age standardized:
  - 28-day emergency admission rates
  - rates of surgery for hernia recurrence

- Emergency admissions to hospitals for people aged over 75 (per 1000 75-year-olds)

- Emergency psychiatric readmission rate

- Infant deaths – a composite indicator consisting of:
  - stillbirth rates
  - infant mortality rates

- Survival rates for breast and cervical cancer – a composite indicator of five-year survival rates consisting of age and sex standardized:
  - survival rates from breast cancer (ages 50–69)
  - survival rates from cervical cancer (ages 15–74)

- Avoidable deaths – a composite indicator of potentially avoidable deaths consisting of:
  - peptic ulcer (ages 25–74)
  - fracture of skull and intracranial injury (ages 1+)
  - maternal deaths (ages 15–44)
  - tuberculosis (ages 5–64)
  - Hodgkin's disease (ages 5–64)
  - chronic rheumatic heart disease (ages 5–44)
  - hypertensive and cerebrovascular disease (ages 35–64)
  - asthma (ages 5–44)
  - appendicitis, abdominal hernia, cholelithiasis and cholecystitis (ages 5–64)
  - coronary heart disease (ages under 65)

Better but not perfect

The list includes indicators for primary care practice and clinical effectiveness, clinical indicators for hospital practice and indicators for health authorities who will be held to account for delivering the whole package. Consultation exercises have already been conducted during 1997 on the clinical and primary care indicators and the 1998 list is also undergoing consultation. This list is not, and never will be, perfect, but significant progress is being made in defining the appropriate products of health care in a comprehensive system. At present, no suitable measures exist for integrated care in the community or for continuing care; this reflects the traditional lack of emphasis on, and information about, these sectors.

Few of the proposed indicators offer anything new although they have not been used to performance-manage health authorities before. Some of the indicators, such as notification rates, are worthless as they have no scientific validity or consistency. Others, such as cervical cancer (survival), cover events which are so rare as to be meaningless over periods of less than 10 years. Nonetheless, unless measures such as these are used to change the way the NHS is managed, no effort will be put into improving the ones now on offer. Necessity may prove to be the mother of invention.

There is full recognition of the poverty of knowledge about what patients want and think. It is intended to carry out a national survey of patient and user experience with analysis of the results possible at individual health authority level. It is not yet known whether it will be possible to differentiate between smaller areas such as those to be covered by primary care groups. There is growing concern among health scientists that this Government, like others, uses statistics to prove what it wants but rejects statistical analysis to explain variations. Most variations at local level are not statistically significant; it would be wrong to change policy on the basis of such findings.

9

How the money will flow: from red tape to patient care

How, not how much?

What should be the crucial chapter for most NHS staff and observers turns out to be the dullest. In the absence of cabinet agreement on the future of NHS funding, all that can be offered is a critique of the old system of distributing funds and an outline of the approach to the new system. The basic problem facing the Government is that the internal market is the means by which funds allocated by Parliament reach the point of expenditure. To replace the internal market, without returning to the monopolies of 1990, has tested the Government's ingenuity. The chosen solution, allocation to primary care groups which then allocate to NHS trusts through long-term agreements, is a reasonable compromise.

Quality, not money, following patients

The key changes have been described in earlier chapters, including unifying budgets in primary care groups, flexible use of these resources, stability through long-term agreements, benchmarking costs of NHS trusts and reducing bureaucracy. Two additional changes are proposed: a new allocation formula which, although not specified at this level, will give greater weight to inner city deprivation; and a revised approach to major capital schemes using the regenerated private finance initiative and putting clinical needs at the top of the criteria list for prioritizing building schemes. The previous Government's reforms sought to ensure that money followed patients in the health system; it worked only up to a point and it stops working when the money runs out. While the underlying principles (freedom of movement for patients and reward for good services) remain valid, penalizing sub-standard performance with financial leverage is to be replaced by mechanisms which raise poor performance so that, in common with the Calman–Hine principles, care of high and even quality is available to all.

Collective responsibility and risk sharing

There is a strong push for the development and value of longer-term agreements and NHS trusts are given a share of the responsibility for ensuring that activity does not get out of kilter with funding, one of the drivers for the current insolvency of the NHS. GPs will continue to have the freedom to refer and to prescribe the drugs which patients need, within the overall budget of the primary care group, but without the bureaucracy of the extra-contractual referral system. How this will be replaced is not yet known, another area where further guidance is awaited and one of the few where it is needed.

More management but at less cost

The drive to reduce expenditure on management and administration has been a cause célèbre of successive governments. NHS management costs go in cycles – rising in 1974, falling in 1982, rising at the end of the 1980s and early 90s and falling again since

1994. The current round of reductions will lead to an overall reduction in management costs as a proportion of total NHS expenditure of the order of 0.7% from 1997 to 2002. The main means of doing so while retaining competent management are outlined in Box 21. It is also believed by many, including politicians, that organizational mergers will release resources from management overheads. This can be an illusion unless the reduction in management costs is a sine qua non for the merger. The belief is likely to be sorely tested during the current frenetic round of mergers.

Box 21   Cutting bureaucracy in *The New NHS*

Ending the internal market will reduce bureaucracy by:

- replacing the annual contracting round with long-term agreements
- abolishing ECRs and cost-per-case contracts
- moving from GP fundholding to inclusive primary care groups
- reshaping health authorities with savings in core administration (independent contractor services) allowing reinvestment in their new role
- ending competition and bearing down on NHS trust management and administrative costs generated by the internal market
- integrating primary care and community trusts
- sharing support functions between NHS organizations

10

Making it happen: rolling out change

An agenda for action

This final chapter lays out the early actions by this Government in implementing changes to the NHS. Early milestones are signalled in Box 22 and actions already taken are described in Box 23. Overall, there is a hint of optimism and a great deal of determination. The believability of the strategy is dented only by the claim that the White Paper will not lead to a wholesale reorganization, when we have already seen that such an outcome is inevitable, due to the radicalism of the proposals as well as the games that NHS managers like to play. The population health targets set by the public health strategy are integrated better with the planning process than *Health of the Nation* could ever be with the internal market. *Our Healthier Nation* is also better focused on primary care which was almost completely bypassed by its predecessor.

HAZ and HAZ-nots

Health Action Zones remain obscure in their uniqueness; do they offer any more than a particular model of multi-agency approaches

Box 22   Early milestones

1998

- Three telephone advice helplines set up (staffed by nurses)
- Projects established to demonstrate the benefits of the NHSnet
- A new Information Management and Technology Strategy for the NHS to be published
- Consultation documents on quality and performance issues
- Public Health Green Paper, *Our Healthier Nation*, issued
- Health Action Zones begin
- A new NHS Charter
- The first national survey of users and carers
- Health authorities begin work with partner organizations on prototype Health Improvement Programmes for 1999
- GP Commissioning Pilots begin
- Development work on primary care groups, on new financial arrangements and on new performance indicators

1999

- Introduction of two-week waiting time limit for urgent suspected breast cancer
- New primary care groups begin, subsuming GP fundholding
- New statutory duties on partnership, health and quality
- Development of local clinical governance, the new National Institute for Clinical Excellence and Commission for Health Improvement
- New unified local health budgets for hospital and community services (commissioning), GP prescribing and the general practice infrastructure
- New funding arrangements for NHS trusts in place

Box 23   Early action on the six key principles

- Action to raise standards across the country in breast cancer services and paediatric care, in a single National Health Service

- Announcement of new Health Action Zones to explore new, flexible, local ways of delivering health and health care

- A new approach to partnership in the NHS for the 1998/99 commissioning round

- Action to improve efficiency by reducing management costs

- Action teams to tackle inherited rising waiting lists and times, improving performance across the country

- Rebuilding public confidence by opening NHS trust board meetings to the public and launching consultation on a new NHS Charter

to health and the integration of health and social care? I understand that the Health Action Zone model will be used initially to provide the framework for major hospital building and restructuring schemes using the private finance initiative, for embracing the wider public health agenda in deprived areas, and as part of local regeneration projects including single regeneration budget proposals and European Union initiatives. I suspect that the approach originally described in the Health Action Zone trailer became adopted as the norm before this White Paper was completed, hence the fairly downbeat presentation of Health Action Zones here. Everyone will be doing it but only a select few will get the badge and the tee-shirt.

Do I perceive realism?

In summary, this is the first long-term structural strategy for the NHS for a quarter of a century. It has many strengths and time to iron out the weaknesses. The biggest obstacle is the full engagement of the professions in the initial structures – where are the incentives? However, the Government does recognize that some changes take time while others will be pushed harder in the short term, a sense of realism which is heartening.

Part 3

Themes for the future

Primary care provision

W(h)ither the independent practitioner

Every reorganization of the NHS brings with it concerns among general practitioners that their independent contractor status is under threat. It has so far survived not only the 50 years of the NHS but also the creation of the NHS itself. The assurances given to general practitioners about the retention of their independence in this White Paper are of uncertain security. It is known that Treasury analysis suggests that the current arrangements for resourcing primary care are not a particularly bad deal for public funding. Despite the natural resistance to private enterprise in the NHS, the independent contractor status has survived successive Labour and Conservative administrations which have done their best to control the professions in many ways. It is certainly possible that this Government will take advantage of its own strength and the lack of opposition to its NHS proposals to have a go at independent contractor status as never before.

The *NHS (Primary Care) Act 1997*, passed by the previous Government, provides a legislative basis on which to initiate pilots involving the direct employment of general practitioners. Further measures have been introduced since the election to allow the employment of GP Principals to address certain service deficiencies and to fill temporary gaps in services to patients. Where recruitment of Principals has traditionally been difficult, due to the excessive cost of buying into expensively propertied practices mainly in inner city areas, direct employment could become a common feature of primary care in both medicine and dentistry.

Primary care trusts hold the key

The new proposals for primary care groups, leading to primary care trust status, offer a wider range of incentives and opportunities for change. By integrating commissioning budgets, prescribing costs and cash-limited GMS funds, and moving towards equalization of primary care funding across the country, more resources will be available for primary care than it is possible to spend under the current system, in areas where recruitment is difficult and list sizes are high. It is more likely that primary care groups will invest these resources in new ways of providing primary care, in order to reduce the burden on themselves, than in adding to secondary care investment. This could be the stimulus to employed Principals as the basis of primary care in cities.

It is also becoming clear that the creation of primary care trusts will provide a systematic opportunity to vary the national GMS contract. While there may be small beginnings, there should be plenty of time under this Government for local contracts to become the norm. While such changes will have to be negotiated, and will presumably be in the interests of local GPs, the benefits for the service as a whole may well eventually justify the buying out of the national contract.

Why change?

There are several reasons to think that the integrated NHS will benefit from changes in the status of GPs. First, primary care trusts will extend primary care as we know it into a continuum including community care and hospitals. The separateness which the independent contractor status gives GPs is a real obstacle to realizing the benefits of integration. It also conferred many advantages but their importance may now be declining while the enormous and growing burden of chronic disease management in the community demands different values and priorities. Second, the White Paper gives a positive boost to the role of nurses in both primary and secondary care. The numbers, status and independence of nurses in primary care in particular are rising; projections are that nursing will become the most numerous profession in primary care within 10 years, even disregarding the community staff employed by NHS trusts. Within the new primary care trusts, nurses will greatly outnumber doctors from the outset. The continued independence of GPs will become increasingly incongruous and the pressure to change will grow.

It may be worth considering whether direct employment of GP Principals actually offers any benefits to the NHS when it is far from obvious that direct employment of hospital consultants for 50 years has rendered them obedient and compliant servants of the State. However, it is likely that an employed primary care workforce would help reduce variations in the availability of primary care across the country through the use of direction of labour. Fifty years of the Medical Practices Committee has failed to achieve this and the present Government is taking equality of access more seriously than any of its predecessors. It may also be argued that the extension of the clinical governance initiative into primary care is going to be toothless unless practitioners are directly employed. The enforcement of clinical and service standards in primary care is critical to the success of the Government's strategy. It should not allow the independent contractor status to sabotage a policy which will have widespread support from the public and other professions; however, all its predecessors have failed in this regard.

Necessity is the mother of invention

In the fullness of time, politics permitting, we can assume that primary care trusts will renegotiate the GMS contract. A recruitment crisis in primary care, now a real possibility, will hasten the acceptability of such a move. The attractiveness of locally negotiated changes to the national contract will lead to the obsolescence and then the redundancy of the Red Book (the statement of fees and allowances which describes the contract between GPs and the Government of the day). The master plan assumes that this will be a voluntary process, with existing practitioners entitled to retain independent contractor status until they retire. Many would probably be persuaded to transfer to employment if they were offered consultant terms and conditions, a guaranteed high salary and security of income.

The last great restrictive practice

There is a major obstacle to the development of primary care along these lines in rural areas. This concerns the rewards received by dispensing practices and the perverse disincentives which the remuneration system currently offers dispensing doctors against cost-efficient prescribing (the practice receives a fixed proportion of the drug cost as a fee, therefore penalizing the practice if it adopts, say, more generic prescribing). This arrangement will have to be renegotiated in a way which protects both the public purse and the continuation of local primary care in rural areas, these smaller practices being dependent on dispensing profits for their economic viability. Conversely, I believe that the integration of prescribing and dispensing provides the ideal model of primary care so long as adequate standards of dispensing practice are met. Eliminating the restrictive practices of dispensing pharmacists may well lead to the decline of the corner shop chemist but, if it leads to integrated primary care, the patient will be the beneficiary.

Health care commissioning

Is it still important?

Commissioning has been the language of the mid-1990s, softening the market jargon of the initial reforms period. Now commissioning is undergoing further change. I believe that the absence of the word 'commissioning' from the title of any of the new structures suggests that it is not as central to the new strategy as might have been expected and less important than the manifesto implied. The key question is whether the primary responsibility of primary care groups is to commission hospital services or to integrate primary and community services provision? While there is no doubt that the budget and the responsibility for commissioning all but the most specialized services will be in the ownership of primary care groups, the determinants of their approach will be the all-embracing Health Improvement Programme and the resource allocation formula.

Collectivism is back

While market disciplines served as the leverage on providers under the terms of the internal market, the new arrangements will be dominated by collective planning and by the performance framework by which all NHS organizations will be held to account. As the medium-term plans are developed and adopted, and as NHS trust performance is tested through benchmarking costs and quality assurance, commissioning will progressively decline in importance.

Farewell to fundholding, welcome partnership

Primary care groups are not the replacement for GP fundholding, nor are they an extension of fundholding to all practices. GP fundholding will be abolished on 31 March 1999 and no decisions on hospital and community health services will be practice-based thereafter. There will be no cost-per-case arrangements, either contractual or extra-contractual, although it remains unclear how ECRs will be replaced without compromising the freedom of referral principle. Service agreements will be similar to long-term block contracts with a focus on quality and effectiveness. The strategic context will be set by health authorities in pursuance of national priorities and requirements. All local agencies, including primary care groups, community health councils, NHS trusts and local authorities, will participate in the development of the Health Improvement Programme and all will abide by it. It is not clear how local authorities will be forced to be partners with traditional enemies – there must be many social services staff who have waited for years to get their own back on general practitioners. This is due largely to the independent contractor status of general practitioners being outside the paradigm of social workers, indeed the whole world of business is alien to the social work paradigm. Nonetheless, while GPs expect social workers and others to drop everything to help them, they will expect to be paid extra for signing a form for the social worker – one can understand how the seeds of enmity are sown. Health and local authorities will have to publish joint investment plans for continuing and community care and primary care groups will have to own these plans. It appears as though the Government would like to integrate health and social services planning/commissioning and it can only control this sufficiently through the NHS. However, to do so would highlight and intensify both political turmoil between central and local government and create some extremely tense issues around charging for services, the mixed economy in social care and the loss of local political accountability for social services. This is the anticipated central government preference and rumour is rife about the imminent policy proposals. Pooled budgets and joint bodies for mental health management may provide the pilot for these arrangements.

In summary, while there may be a medium-term future for the joint commissioning of services at the health and social care interface, and the commissioning of specialist health care by primary care groups may be a temporary spur to developing service integration in the next three years, I do not believe that health care commissioning will play a major role in the future of the NHS.

The provision of secondary care in hospitals

Reconfiguring NHS trusts

The existing configuration of NHS trusts is an unstructured network of community trusts, mental health trusts, learning disabilities trusts, acute hospitals trusts, combinations of any two, three or four of these and specialist trusts occupying part of a hospital. There are also specialist ambulance services trusts. Various mergers are taking place, mostly of like with like, and mixed trusts are being reconfigured along specialist or geographical lines. Vertical and horizontal integration is reducing the number of trusts but making no more sense than the original. The proposals in the White Paper will radically change the configuration of NHS trusts.

Community health services will be transferred to primary care trusts; mental health and learning disabilities services will be separated from acute general hospital services where they are now combined and will be provided exclusively by specialist providers in order to sustain quality, develop specialization and reduce the risk of service failures leading to homicides; existing combined services trusts will be reduced in size as they become reduced to general hospitals only and they will come under pressure to merge. As the pressure to reduce management costs builds, and community services are transferred, the number of remaining NHS trusts must reduce too in order to spread the management overheads. The medical Royal Colleges are making recommendations for the future organization of hospital services which would operate on a much larger basis than the 250 000 population which was the guide for the development of the district general hospital. In future, NHS hospital trusts are likely to cover population catchments of at least 500 000.

The future configuration of providers will be based on primary care trusts, specialist mental health/learning disabilities trusts and large general hospital trusts. Excluding primary care trusts, the total number of NHS trusts may fall from over 450 at the beginning of 1998, to about 200 during the next four years.

More doctors but fewer beds

Larger hospital trusts will have much bigger teams of clinicians, perhaps working in more than one hospital and meeting Royal College requirements for sub-specialization. Bigger teams with more specialists can develop tertiary service provision and the traditional district general hospital will cease to be universal. Future hospital models will include teaching hospitals, large general hospitals with some specialist services, and small local hospitals offering a limited range of specialties.

The drive for greater efficiency in the hospital service will continue to put pressure on hospital bed numbers. Only the bigger hospitals will have the flexibility to survive.

The commissioning and provision of specialist services

Come back region, (almost) all is forgiven

Before the 1991 reforms, a wide range of specialist services, including dialysis, radiotherapy, transplantation, cardiac surgery, genetics services and neurosciences, were planned and funded by regional health authorities. These responsibilities transferred to district health authorities in most cases; this has resulted in both fragmentation of the commissioning of services and complexity for their providers. During the last two years, health authorities have attempted to adopt collective approaches to the commissioning of these tertiary services to reduce their risk and the risk to the integrity of the services, often the fastest growing areas of hospital care, at the leading edge of technology, frequently emotive and often undergoing evaluation rather than of proven benefit. These moves, which are by no means universal, have generally been regarded as successful and the White Paper gives to NHS Executive Regional Offices the responsibility for ensuring that such arrangements are in place everywhere and operate effectively.

Precedents exist

Various supra-regional service commissioning arrangements exist for services such as liver transplantation and complex cranio-facial surgery which are provided by one provider for more than one region. The high-security psychiatric services commissioning board (for the special hospitals) and the national specialist commissioning advisory group fulfil these responsibilities and the services are funded through a national levy on all health authorities. These arrangements appear to work well in controlling costs, preventing creepage in service provision, maintaining the quality of services and ensuring fair and equal access based only on clinical need. However, they represent only 10% of these highly specialized services by cost and regionally based services do not enjoy this systematic approach, access is unfair – heavily biased towards the populations which are situated close to the specialist providers – and there is a lack of specialist services commissioning expertise in health authorities.

The services and the funding

Such services (*see* Box 24 for examples), which tend to be small in volume and high in unit cost, can be funded through top-slicing – an equitable levy on the health authorities concerned – or through bottom-slicing – individual investment contributions offered by each authority, usually inequitably. The latter method, favoured by the internal market, does not result in equal access related to clinical need as health authorities face these services with different levels of affordability and variable positions among their own priorities. Many authorities favour their local providers and regard investment in specialist providers outside their own areas as undesirable although these services may offer excellent clinical value. As leading-edge clinical services tend to be fast-growing, the tension between meeting justified clinical need and affordability can be very high. Some authorities tend to be isolationist and would rather commission these types of services from their own providers even though they may not possess the skills required; quality assurance is one of the principal aims of collective commissioning and one of the first victims of fragmentation.

> **Box 24   Examples of specialist regional services**
>
> - Neurosurgery and specialist neurology
> - Cardiac surgery and highly specialized cardiology
> - Radiotherapy and specialist oncology
> - Bone marrow transplantation
> - Clinical genetics services
> - Neonatal intensive care
> - Paediatric intensive care
> - Specialist adult intensive care (neuro, cardiac, multi-system failure)
> - Acute renal failure services
> - Renal transplantation and dialysis services
> - Brain injury rehabilitation
> - Medium-secure psychiatric care
> - Haemophilia services
> - Cystic fibrosis care
> - Specialist burns care
> - Spinal injuries
> - Cochlear implantation

Partnership again

The population base for these services is over one million, sometimes many more, larger than almost all health authorities and therefore requiring multi-authority approaches. As the only expert knowledge about these services resides in the providers themselves, they too need to be involved in the planning process. Only in this way can the confidence of providers, especially the clinicians, in the process be assured. The services involved, such as bone marrow transplantation and clinical genetics, are not only among the fastest-growing health services, they are of potentially very high added value. They are best developed, supported and utilized effectively through top-sliced funding arrangements. As these reforms are implemented, the restructuring of health authorities and the redrawing of their boundaries may well be based on the catchment areas for these highly specialized services, to integrate their commissioning at the level of the populations serviced. However, the commissioning expertise will not be based in health authorities in the future; they will be strategic organizations and primary care groups will employ the commissioning staff. Specialist providers will recoil in horror at the prospect of having to deal with up to 25 primary care groups; their experience with fundholders, not necessarily representative of the future, will have shown them that small commissioners think small – these services require vision and overview. The development of specialist commissioning units for these services, at regional office, multi-authority or individual authority level is possible but in all cases the providers must be involved. A more rational model would be to integrate the commissioning and the provision of some of these services, such as specialized mental health services, with a regional commissioning board representing health authorities and primary care groups to oversee balance and affordability. This would be an example of true vertical integration within a specialist NHS trust, a model which might work for specialist mental health services too.

A consultation paper published in April 1998 seeks views on these and related options and envisages a three-year implementation plan commencing in 1999.

Changes in NHS structure and new roles for new and old organizations

What's in a name?

The names may be the same but the shape, size and role of all NHS organizations is shortly to change. Some of the changes are early and are required to deliver the primary agenda; others will emerge later and will be a consequence of the initial actions. All are probable and most are inevitable.

THE NHS EXECUTIVE

Still in charge

The NHS Executive and its Regional Offices will continue to be the managerial top of the NHS. There is more than a hint of growing tension between the Executive and the rest of the Department of Health, with a possibility – no stronger than that – of their merger in a few years when these reforms are worked through. In the meantime, the Executive, especially in the regions, will take more control over planning, performance management of health authorities, the new commissioning responsibilities for regional services and quality assurance, e.g. of national screening programmes. The Health Improvement Programmes and the national performance framework will be the key tools of control for the Executive and, as the future of Regional Offices becomes more uncertain, they will become increasingly difficult to work with and they will lose sight of the overall aims of the White Paper changes. The central NHS Executive is energetically engaged in attempting to control the implementation of the White Paper; this is what government departments do, however undesirable, unnecessary or pointless. The changes will occur despite them and they will be driven by health authorities themselves and not by guidance. Contrary to popular belief, most NHS managers thrive on action and especially that generated by re-organizations. Since health authorities have known for some time that the previous Government's reforms were sinking in a swamp of bickering and bureaucracy, they are filled with enthusiasm and energy for any suitable alternative such as the proposals in *The New NHS*.

Cuts on the horizon

As the changes bed down, after primary care trusts are created and NHS trusts are reconfigured, health authorities will merge and the whole Executive structure will have to be revisited. Under the present arrangements, health authorities and NHS trusts are accountable to separate divisions in each regional office. These divisions should merge in 1998 to produce a unified performance management function. Increasingly, Health Improvement Programmes will be representative of all local NHS bodies, including both health authorities and NHS trusts. Joint account-ability through the HIP will become the norm with *de facto* horizontal integration of local NHS trusts and health authorities.

Within three or so years, the number of organizations (health authorities and NHS trusts) being monitored will have been cut by half. It is likely that the number of Regional Offices will be cut and they may be abolished altogether if health authorities are deemed big enough and sufficiently competent to take on the new regional responsibilities for specialist services commissioning. An area of uncertainty concerns the continuing separation between the health and social care sides of the Department of Health. If the Govern-ment is committed to integrating health and social care policy, is it going to consider integrating the top of the office too?

HEALTH AUTHORITIES

Tried and trusted or no alternative?

In England, there are currently 100 health authorities and they are responsible for allocating resources and picking up the pieces. They are expected to manage an internal market which does not work with few sanctions and little leverage and no co-ordination of other purchasers, especially fundholders. Since May 1997, their powers over fundholders have gradually increased, including the ability to reclaim budgets to handle emergency pressures. From April 1998, they acquire the primary responsibility for establishing the new structures, especially primary care groups. They are also taking the lead in proposing and delivering reconfiguration of services in NHS trusts, based mainly on service needs, especially the inte-gration of specialist acute services, but also driven by the need to deliver savings in management costs. Further action is likely to release savings from improving the uses of the NHS estate, much of which is owned by NHS trusts but some of which, mainly closed mental hospitals, is vested in the Secretary of State. Health authorities will have to lead this work as NHS trusts have vested interests.

Planning returns

The new health authorities will be gradually giving up their commissioning functions during 1999 and beyond to primary care groups, except for the remaining specialist services. From summer 1998, health authorities will have to establish an inclusive planning system for the production of the first Health Improvement Programme in April 1999. This initial plan will probably be an advanced draft rather than the fully developed three- to five-year plan which will eventually be required. The HIP will be substantially influenced by the public health White Paper expected towards the end of 1998 and will focus on population-level benefits in terms of health action and health gain from health care in the national priority target areas (expected to be heart disease and stroke, cancer, accidents and suicide). Planning is not a highly developed function in the NHS as it has been out of favour for 10 years. Even before the Thatcher revolution took firm hold in the late 1980s, health service strategic planning was weak, lacking in vision and almost devoid of implementation. Now, a service which has rejected planning as a discipline for a decade, has to deliver the most ambitious and broadly based plan ever required. This is a tall order under any circumstances; to do so in the midst of structural destabilization is well nigh impossible. However, as one Minister was heard to say to their most senior civil servant, failure is not acceptable.

Leading on clinical effectiveness

In addition to the reincarnation and improvement of planning, health authorities will be establishing their leadership role in implementing clinical effectiveness. Most authorities have gone through a period of maturity during the last seven years since the market and the NHS R&D strategy began. Initially, it was thought that the contracting process would be the means by which changes in practice would be achieved. Then it was realized that contracts were merely pieces of paper which nobody read and that changes in practice required more positive action such as sanctions (usually fines) for non-compliance and threats to transfer services. Latterly, it has dawned on all but the most stupid that the old ways were best; that change in practice resulted from partnership and mutual benefit not from antagonism and threats. This is the stage reached with most health authorities and trusts. There remain consultants, even in well-motivated trusts, who resist the idea of change and especially that which makes them like other people. However, most doctors regard effective health care and clinical audit as helpful disciplines, their only argument being when the zealots pursue the principles of clinical effectiveness further than is valid. Other professions have generally been more positive and are keen to participate, although some professions have no knowledge base on which to defend much of what they do. These processes work best when they are internalized by the organizations concerned. The leadership role of health authorities is a throwback to the market mentality; leadership must come from the professions at local level if change is to be achieved. I would suggest that the health authority role is to support and promote and develop internal leadership in NHS trusts and primary care groups and not to impose or pontificate. Thanks to the NHS R&D strategy, the knowledge base to underpin this work is growing and is freely accessible electronically. The use of the evidence in National Service Frameworks and by the National Institute of Clinical Excellence means that no local organization needs to possess its own intelligence function, merely the means to access the products of others. What we do not want is every health authority building a department of clinical effectiveness which sets out to tell clinicians what to do; we should be beyond that stage by now.

Strange bedfellows

One of the more daunting tasks facing health authorities is the engagement of local authorities in the new planning and public health approach. The structural political distance between the (central government) NHS and (locally democratic) local authorities has been a barrier to effective joint working since the end of the Second World War. The scope of interest of local government has been progressively reduced and restricted to their statutory responsibilities, and the financial pressures facing them have persuaded counsellors to ignore the majority of other matters including health. The structure of local authorities and their responsibilities does not lend itself the opportunity to handle health; it is handled, as in much of the NHS, in its component parts, e.g. environment, social services, leisure (also non-statutory). Now, local authorities are faced with a statutory duty to share responsibility for health and social care planning with the NHS and, in the eyes of some observers, are poised to lose some of their role for social care. A further White Paper on social care is expected soon and will throw light on the Government's intentions but a sense of destabilization and insecurity is deeply felt among social services staff. This does not provide the most auspicious setting for a renewal of joint ownership of health issues; nonetheless, local authorities are under as much pressure as health authorities to succeed in this venture. Unlike health authorities, however, local authorities are not accountable to central government but to their own electorate; a neat conundrum for the Government.

NHS trusts: no longer quite so self-governing

In addition to these new powers and responsibilities, health authorities are to be given new reserve powers over the exercise of responsibilities by NHS trusts. These will include the overview of estate utilization referred to earlier and also to expenditure on capital schemes and, perhaps most important of all, control over new consultant appointments. One of the most important reasons for the insolvency of the NHS, and especially in local pockets of the country, is the rise in the number of consultants and other medical staff. Doctors and hospital beds are the key supply side factors in driving up demand for specialist care. Some NHS trusts increased their consultant staffing so quickly, often without reference to the needs of commissioners, that house prices were affected upwards in those areas. In future, all such changes will have to be approved by health authorities and funding will have to be collectively agreed by the trust, health authority and primary care group(s).

NHS TRUSTS

The jury is out

In the 1991 reforms, NHS trusts were the vanguard of culture change, the paradigm shifters who would permanently change the behaviour of the health professions and the health industry. Gradually they have become the victims of their own rhetoric and of sometimes perverse market-style purchasing by fundholders which has resulted in sporadic disinvestment and some resource transfer to the private sector. Whether the market has led to increased efficiency and improved quality is not clear, partly because there were no formal experiments or evaluation and partly because the changes observed since 1991 were mostly continuations of trends established during the previous decade. The scene looks better and clearer from the fundholders perspective, where improvements in primary care and some improvements in services for patients are apparent. We have already seen how the freedoms of NHS trusts are being slightly restricted so that more decisions have to be agreed in advance by health authorities. They will retain, for the time being, freedoms in terms of pay and terms and conditions though these may well be eroded in the future.

Partnership and quality

NHS trusts will continue to be freestanding organizations with their own boards and corporate governance. They will be the providers of specialist hospital and specialist mental health services, and initially the employers of community health staff also, and will plan the future of these services in partnership with health authorities and primary care groups. To reinforce this behaviour, they will have a new statutory duty of partnership (with health authorities) and a statutory duty for quality (of clinical care). These duties are subject to legislation and their precise meaning and purpose is not yet clear. The other major challenge to NHS trusts is the introduction of the concept of clinical governance.

Publicly accountable

Under the terms of the internal market, NHS trusts were accountable to their purchasers through contracts and to the NHS Executive for their statutory duties, all financial. Given the dissatisfaction with the internal market and the widespread insolvency, this could not be regarded as a successful mechanism. Under the new arrangements, the costs of NHS trusts will be compared with reference costs for procedures published nationally by the Department of Health. Although the White Paper does not specifically state that the costs of individual NHS trusts will be published, it is highly likely that this will be a game that the media will play. (The schools league tables were an invention of the Sunday papers, not of the previous Government.) It can reasonably be assumed therefore that NHS trusts will be held to account in public for variations in their procedure costs and that any costs above the average will be (perhaps correctly) branded as waste. They will also be held to account indirectly for their contributions to the joint Health Improvement Programme, although the formal process will focus on the accountability of health authorities. A NHS trust which is failing to perform adequately will come under the review of the Commission for Health Improvement (CHIMP). It is also possible that other failing structures, in terms of efficiency, effectiveness or partnership, including health authorities and primary care groups may be similarly challenged although the details are not yet clear. The Secretary of State has proposed that (s)he retains reserve powers to dispose of the boards of NHS trusts which are not performing to the required standard. Such a move would probably only occur after a particularly damaging report by CHIMP. These arrangements reflect those now operating for schools and, in that example, the reserve powers have been used.

Overworked, overpaid and overstressed

Although working in a much more managed environment than hitherto, NHS trusts remain the mainstay of specialist health care with many of their freedoms still intact. The return to partnership working will not be a problem for many NHS staff, including senior managers, although the much higher salaries paid to trust executive directors, compared with their health authority colleagues, may cause local tension.

The future of most NHS trust executives (and non-executives) is in the balance, however, as inevitable changes in trust configuration start to bite. Between 1997 and 2000, most NHS trusts will merge or undergo major restructuring. The reasons (*see* Box 25) are universal and unavoidable and will lead to a reduction of over a half in the total number of NHS trusts.

Box 25 Triggering factors for NHS trust reconfiguration

- Transfer of community services to primary care trusts (Tier 4)

- Transfer of community hospitals to primary care trusts (Tier 4)

- Mental health and learning disabilities services to be managed by specialist providers

- Continued bearing down on NHS trust management costs

- Medical Royal College recommendations on the organization of medical and surgical specialties for populations of 500 000

- The need to change the culture of NHS trusts to facilitate the new duty of partnership

- Tackling recurring deficits in NHS trusts

PRIMARY CARE GROUPS

Pulling together

GP fundholders are either leaders or followers; the leaders are consonant, believe in the principles of fundholding, campaign for the retentions of its freedoms and flexibility and vigorously defend its advantages; the followers are dissonant, are uncomfortable with the principles, became fundholders because the option of not doing so was threatening to them and their patients and are content with the prospect of a return to a more collective approach to local service planning. Non-fundholders are also of two types; some reject the principles so profoundly that they have declined all pressure and incentive to join the scheme; others are simply disconnected from the world of the NHS market and never saw the need to become involved. The only real problem is that all these types of GP are now expected to work together for the mutual benefit of all their patients in primary care groups.

A new start

In all respects, primary care groups are new organizations, not a replacement for fundholding or the extension of total purchasing pilot projects. They are collective, geographical arrangements of community and primary care staff, led initially by GPs and community nurses. They will both provide services and commission them, the vertical integration enjoyed by district health authorities prior to the reforms of the previous Government enhanced by the horizontal integration of the first contact services including housing and social care. They look very much like a transitional arrangement between the era of the internal market with the primary care-led NHS and the independence of the small business in health, and the age of collectivism in a modern society. In this latter vision, people and organizations work together for a common good but in a manner which is subject to external review and contestability, where good performance is rewarded and poor performance is not tolerated. This is a noble and ambitious goal and not one which has ever been achieved in peacetime, and only exceptionally in wartime, by English-speaking peoples.

Managing primary care

Two important features of primary care groups are not yet fully worked through. First, they are accountable to health authorities for their delivery of the Health Improvement Programme but are they equally accountable as providers? The active management of primary care is the one missing element in all previous NHS structures; these proposals provide, for the first time, an appropriate framework for peer-led management of general medical services and related primary care and community services. Second, local democracy continues to be excluded from the NHS although local elected members (of local authorities) are likely to have an increased presence on the boards of NHS trusts and health authorities, though in the latter case possibly in competition with their own chief executives. It is possible that the ultimate manifestation of primary care groups and trusts will be a locally democratic body, providing true local public accountability for any part of the health service for the first time since 1974.

Sized for integrating service delivery

The proposed size of primary care groups, at around 100 000 population, is arbitrary. It is bigger than any practice and bigger than almost all total purchasing pilots, but smaller than all health authorities. They are therefore unlike any existing structure in size and will necessitate new partnerships and relationships to be forged. If service commissioning were the main task of primary care groups, the proposed size would be pointless; it has been demonstrated in other countries, e.g. Netherlands, that a population of at least one million is required for effective commissioning. Of course, it is possible that the British Government is adopting pointless policies; it would not be the first time. However, I believe that commissioning is not the main agenda but integration of primary, community and social care is. A community of 100 000 may be an appropriate basis for service integration. However, the management cost burden will be higher at this size than with larger groups and it must be on the cards for primary care groups to merge at about the time that they aspire to primary care trust status. This would bring them up to the average size of a district health authority before 1991 (c. 250 000).

Social tension

The prospects for integrating social care into this framework are somewhat remote at the present time. Local authority social services have had a trying time in recent years in terms of scandals, funding and priorities. The usually hysterical and self-righteous public and political reaction to service failures by social workers has not abated under new Ministers. It is of course tragic when people under care or supervision are abused or killed but the nature of the work and the clients requires some risks to be taken and some failures are inevitable. The culture of blaming does a disservice to social work professionals and is also dishonest to the community, implying that all service failures are avoidable and that therefore someone must be blamed. The transfer of social services to non-political accountability is unlikely to be acceptable but the desire for service integration of care of the elderly and mentally ill is strong enough for some bold moves. It is, for example, possible for all children's services in local authorities to be integrated into a single department, including education and child protection. It is probable that mental health services and budgets will be integrated in some experimental pilot projects. The real challenge comes with elderly care, the biggest slice of both health and social care, and the main target for primary and community care integration.

The paradox of practice-level change

Perhaps the greatest challenge of all for primary care groups is the marriage of collectivism and the achievement of improvements at practice level. While the end of fundholding will abolish routine practice-level collection of commissioning data, it is precisely these data which will be required to stimulate behaviour change in the use of specialist services and in securing effective service integration. The management resources available to primary care groups will not be sufficient to support this if downward pressure on management costs continues to excite politicians. A nice paradox for the next Secretary of State!

The renewal of health care planning

Rediscovery

A consensus approach to health service planning was introduced into local levels of the NHS in 1975. Capital and strategic planning had been an integral part of hospital administration from the beginning of the NHS. Neither process was altogether successful but NHS staff were involved in the system and they had faith in it. Planning is incompatible with a market-driven economy which is based on choices made by purchasers and providers; such choices are distorted by planning. The market philosophy of the Thatcher years led to the decline of planning in public services and was informally dropped from the health service management system in 1991.

No market, no plans, no chance

As the NHS reforms were implemented, planners became contractors and commissioners of care. Although the reforms led to service changes, especially through fundholding, a market did not really exist as it was overmanaged by the NHS Executive and political considerations protected the weak from market disciplines and consequences. A service without planning and relatively protected from market rules is uncontrolled and undirected. Providers grew on clinical whim; NHS trusts developed into niche markets for which they were ill-equipped, which proved to be illusions and could not be afforded; and small purchasers transferred contracts for personal rather than objective reasons. The resulting service is fragmented, overexpanded, insolvent, unsustainable and ready for change.

The cancer model

Amid this growing chaos, the Chief Medical Officers of England and Wales (Kenneth Calman and Deirdre Hine) attempted something unusually bold in the midst of John Major's conservative administration; they published a model centralist plan for cancer services which was so good that even the Government had to accept it. The health service found various ways of implementing the eponymous report and found that it liked planning and that health services benefited as a result. Thanks to the Calman–Hine report, the NHS has rediscovered the joys of planning, the relationships it forges, the horizontal and vertical integration and the unifying goals of better health care for both managers and clinicians. The proposed National Service Frameworks are based on the Calman–Hine approach which uses evidence-based approaches to complex planning issues and enables rational planning for services to patients which cross many sectors of care and several tiers of services. A list of proposed services to be handled in this way will be issued shortly; the approach will encourage a patient-focused model of services leading to commissioned programmes of care.

Action in zones

A further planning initiative launched by the Government is the establishment of Health Action Zones to promote innovative approaches to public health and community care initiatives, especially in deprived city areas. These initiatives are part of the overarching Government strategy to reduce social exclusion. However, while similar initiatives in other Government departments, such as Education Action Zones, are labels to be avoided and are small scale (a pyramid of 5 to 20 schools), Health Action Zones are sought after prizes and large scale (at least as big as a health authority).

Programme planning

The all-inclusive Health Improvement Programmes, co-ordinated by health authorities, will constitute the medium-term plan for health and health care in the area. Commissioning plans of primary care groups and the business plans of NHS trusts will follow the HIP. Planning, not purchasing, is the language of *The New NHS*. The distribution of funds will follow the implementation of the Health Improvement Programme, including joint plans with social services for continuing and community care from April 1999. Children's services plans, currently the responsibility of social services, could also be included in this framework at a later date.

Skills and culture required

The package of planning initiatives sets the scene for the long-term development of national and local health services, driven by a strategy to promote the health of populations. However, some important requirements for successful planning have not been addressed. NHS planning skills were never the best and many have been lost to the NHS during the last seven years. The existing proposals assume a professional planning process with an inclusive approach to health professions and other organizations. However, the NHS still does not have a systematic mechanism for involving the public in decision-making. Community health councils, established as part of the NHS reorganization in 1974 and a sop to the immature consumerism of the era, have largely failed to represent the public, tending to fall between the stools of minority lobbying and seduction by health authorities. The CHCs receive scant attention in the White Paper; only one mention in passing and no clear role established. They might well have been abolished in earlier reorganizations but were presumably not regarded as sufficiently important to bother with. Local authorities are representative of local people and, frequently, regard themselves as the only surviving vestiges of electoral accountability. Their lack of responsibility for health services has not prevented many local authorities from launching interest groups, concerned as much with the unaccountability of the NHS as with health policy itself. Given the low turnout at local elections, and the incompatibility between local authority rhetoric and actions, such initiatives have, in their most extreme manifestations, been hypocritical, expensive and pointless. The new role for local authorities in health requires a mature and engaged approach which will require a new local political will and some time to bed down. The continuing democratic deficit, notwithstanding the insincerity of previous local authority actions, is something which has yet to be addressed. It will be interesting to see the intentions of a government whose ardour for regional government has cooled somewhat since the narrowness of the Welsh referendum, while still flirting with lesser symbols of devolution such as elected mayors and posing experimental models for government such as replacing committees with focus groups.

Research and development and clinical effectiveness

Beyond research

The maturing R&D strategy and the shifted focus towards implementing effective health care is a logical and welcomed approach. The previous Government was genuinely enthusiastic about R&D for the NHS, presumably based on the Treasury's belief that it could lead to reduced expenditure. The new Government, while not necessarily having the same delusions, does believe in the intrinsic rectitude of doing the right things, i.e. clinical effectiveness. The evidence is clear that effective care improves clinical outcomes and that comparative evidence can stimulate improvements in efficiency. While there is still a place for primary and secondary research for the NHS, the research budget has been cut and an investment shift towards dissemination of research findings, implementation of effective practice and accountability for effective clinical care (through clinical governance) has been signalled.

Co-ordination, sanctions and incentives

The management of research and development, dissemination, implementation, clinical effectiveness, commissioning of R&D and research provision is totally fragmented. There has been relatively little focus on primary care, despite the largest single research investment by the R&D Directorate (£15 million over 10 years in the National Primary Care Research and Development Centre, based in the Universities of Manchester, Salford and York), little investment in information about primary care provision (unlike secondary care commissioned by primary care) and still no sanctions to apply to deviant practices. Financial incentives have worked modestly in changing primary care practice in prescribing but only at practice level. The new structures require collective commissioning and accountability but practice-level changes in behaviour; the incentives to do this have not yet been invented.

No hiding place

The White Paper proposals provide a systematic framework for the management and accountability for improving the effectiveness of clinical practice (*see* Box 26). At the heart of this framework are the three new pillars of the National Institute for Clinical Excellence (*see* Box 18), National Service Frameworks and the Commission for Health Improvement. Sandwiched by the R&D strategy and increasing professional regulation, the day is approaching when these bodies will expose unprofessional behaviour as never before and the relative protection enjoyed by the medical, and some other, professions when confronted with unjustifiable clinical behaviour is under increasing pressure and will eventually break. The timescale may be long, however, as the National Institute is likely to be located under the auspices of the Academy of Medical Royal Colleges. The Commission, a statutory body operating at arm's length from government, will publish information on the comparative performance of NHS trusts in relation to all three dimensions of quality: effectiveness (health outcomes), equity (access to services) and humanity (patients' and carers' views). This is effectively an extension of the Audit Commission's work into the clinical arena at individual level.

Box 26 The national framework for clinical effectiveness

- The generation of knowledge through primary research (new knowledge) and secondary research (overviews and analyses of existing knowledge) through the NHS R&D Programme

- Establishing programmes of care for important clinical conditions which are based on reliable evidence of effectiveness through National Service Frameworks

- Developing and disseminating clinical service guidelines and audit tools, which are based on reliable findings, by the National Institute for Clinical Excellence

- Overseeing the effectiveness and efficiency of health organizations, including the adoption of the principles of clinical governance, by the Commission for Health Improvement

- Improving clinical practice and internalizing the principles of effective health care and clinical governance through greater self-regulation by the health professions

---

Cost-effectiveness and rationing

The consistent use of the term 'cost-effectiveness' throughout the White Paper suggests that the Government has a lot of friends who are health economists. The absence of a universal database of relative costs and effectiveness limits the value to which the principles and philosophy can be put. However, the will to pursue these values is important. Cost-effectiveness analysis inevitably leads to choices; every choice involves a sacrifice and, where health care is concerned, the sacrifice is what most people would call rationing. Limiting access to services on the basis of effectiveness evidence is now well established in the NHS; limiting access on the basis of a treatment being effective but less cost-effective is more contentious. This is the debate which the Government has opened.

Clinical governance

Quality in clinical practice

After a long and sometimes painful gestation, NHS trusts have given birth to effective clinical practice. This forms the basis of the clinical governance initiative, which could not be imposed on an unwilling health community without the sort of turmoil which met the previous Government's reforms; a few supportive zealots, a host of vigorous opposition and a substantial level of apathy, hoping it will go away. The main characteristics of clinical govern-ance were outlined in Box 14. NHS trusts have to embrace the concept of clinical governance so that quality is at the core of the organization and of every individual health professional.

Accounting for quality

Now that NHS trusts will have a statutory duty for the quality of care they provide, and the chief executive is legally and ultimately responsible for quality of care, formal arrangements will have to be established to enable the Trust Board to be assured that their responsibility for quality of care is being met. This will be through an arrangement similar to that suggested in the White Paper, a sub-committee of the Board headed by a senior professional. In almost all cases, the senior professional will be a consultant; either another job for the trust medical director or another board-level post for a doctor. The clinical governance sub-committee will be responsible for ensuring that the Board's requirements for ensuring internal clinical governance will be fulfilled. It will be necessary to engage clinical staff at every ward, clinic and department and to submit monthly reports on quality to the Board, possibly in public, and to produce an annual report. While, in theory, this regime will put clinical governance on the same level as financial control, trust boards know what they are doing with finance and what to expect; the same will not be true of clinical governance for some time. Firm leadership will be necessary and, for all lead professionals, a good deal of training in handling colleagues, data and the Board. Work has already begun on developing clinical governance training for boards and a rather obscure consultation exercise on clinical governance, presumably seeking a definition, has also been initiated.

Getting to the heart of it

Many NHS trust clinical staff have become accustomed to peer review via clinical audit. There remain a minority who are resistant, often the most senior consultants and an unacceptable proportion of surgeons, though not – it must be stated – their Royal College. The clinical governance agenda is much more penetrating, requiring all professionals to be involved and making clear to the Board those who resist. The only safe strategy for the professions is to embrace the new culture and to co-operate with changes in practice, even when it is their own which is indicated. It is the universality of clinical governance which constitutes its greatest challenge and the openness which gives it its greatest lever.

Clinical governance in primary care

Clinical audit is well established in primary care although it is not universal and is not mandatory except for some chronic disease management packages. Many GPs and their practice staff are actively involved in clinical audit and the prescribing initiative has provided comparative audit for all practices since 1991. However, the greatest variations in practice occur within partnerships and these are not obvious in routine data available to health authorities. It must be assumed that no more precise data will be available to primary care groups. The adoption of clinical governance in primary care groups will focus on primary care behaviour including prescribing, referrals to specialists and clinical care in the practice. It will also cover the indicators of effectiveness in clinical care which form part of the national performance framework (*see* Box 20). The great weakness is that we know so little about what happens in primary care consultations and there is so little evidence of the encounters. I remain unconvinced that much progress will be achieved in improving primary care provision without radical change in the status of the participants.

Mental health: another challenge

Although not quite as ill-prepared as the primary care professions, mental health services face major challenges in adopting clinical governance. The disempowering culture of mental health services has reduced in recent years but significant problems still exist in mental health professions. Applying the basic principles of effective, evidence-based care and outcomes assessment to psychiatry, psychology and psychiatric nursing poses real challenges. There is no prospect of the necessary data being available to monitor the effectiveness of mental health care due to weaknesses in both the diagnostic and therapeutic regimes for mental health. While the academic psychiatric community expend more and more energy on the intellectual, but practically useless, refinement of diagnostic criteria, there is little reliable evidence of what works best and almost no consistency in treatment approaches. There is not much of a framework for CHIMP to assess against.

Whence professional leadership?

Despite the lack of a corporate structure, each primary care group will nominate a senior professional, again presumably a doctor though not specified as such, to take a lead in setting and monitoring clinical service standards and instituting professional development programmes. This will be a substantial task of immense sensitivity and there does not appear to be an obvious basis on which to select the lead professional. Bold volunteers and structured training will be early necessities. To become primary care trusts, groups will have to be able to demonstrate that they have in place systematic monitoring and development of clinical standards in each practice. To proceed with the principles of clinical governance at practice level, a more voluntary approach in each practice is expected. A professional member of each practice will be encouraged to accept lead responsibility for standards and performance; special sensitivity and arrangements for small practices will be required. The potential benefits for patients of these principles could well be substantial and they will be worth waiting for. Forcing rapid change on an unprepared primary care community could do more damage than it is worth. Nurturing and support will be better strategies than demands and formal accountability. Intelligent and altruistic lay involvement may also be a powerful ally.

Towards a definition and a framework

Clinical governance, like R&D before it, will endure long after the new NHS structures pass into oblivion. It will evolve into a combination of developmental initiatives, exemplified by continuous improvement in practice and the creation of a working environment in which excellence can flourish and control systems, especially legal accountability for quality and measures to safeguard standards. The trick is to ensure that the professional focus on development satisfies the political and managerial need for control.

Part 4

The future for the National Health Service

Viability of the new structures

The safety and security of primary care groups and trusts

Assuming a population base of 100 000 and average hospital and prescribing costs, the typical primary care group will have a budget of over £50 million. This will include approximately £40 million for hospital and community health services, £10 million for prescribing costs in primary care and about £2 million for non-cash-limited GMS funding. The management costs of the primary care group will be £300 000 but this will rise to nearer £750 000 after trust status is granted due to the management costs of community services. This is a big enough budget for most uncertainties to be accommodated although recent prescribing cost overruns have embarrassed the whole NHS. (£80 million of the £300 million winter pressures money in 1997/98 was used to cover an overspend on non-fundholders prescribing costs in-year.) Doubling the size of the groups will increase the budget, reduce the proportions spent on management costs, limit the financial risk and raise the scale of primary care trusts to that of former district health authorities, a tried and tested level of accountability. At either size, primary care organizations are unlikely to be coterminous with local authorities. The necessary integration of primary and community care with aspects of social care will be hindered by fragmented boundaries with social care structures; given the Government's priority for this goal, the possibility of formally transferring some aspects of social care commissioning or provision to primary care trusts is genuine.

Changing times for NHS trusts

We are already seeing the frenetic merger activity among NHS trusts to preserve viability and to reduce management costs. These mergers are usually being driven by the need to change service shape in the context of changing standards in clinical service organization. These trends towards increasing specialization and scale of enterprise are going to continue, leading to further pressures on trusts to merge. As NHS trusts grow in size, they will cease to be local organizations; this is bound to cause sensitivities with local communities, as will the redistribution of services which the larger trusts will necessitate. The new NHS trusts will be large and secure but they will also be controversial. While primary care trusts will be local organizations and NHS trusts will be increasingly remote, there may be a move to reintegrate provision or, alternatively, to integrate large NHS trusts with equally large health authorities. Vertical integration of NHS bodies is inevitable at some time in the future, though not necessarily under this Government's 10-year horizon, when all other horizontal integrations have failed to deliver the Holy Grail of higher quality, seamless care, declining costs and public popularity. It may be worth preparing early!

Temporary leadership for health authorities

The new health authorities will have a limited but strategic role. Strategy implies long term and this should be sufficient to give health authorities the status they require to lead. However, relieved of their commissioning and primary care administrative functions, the existing authorities will become small organizations, too small to be truly strategic. The real purpose of health authorities is to establish the new structures, then, as happened to regional health authorities in 1994, having rendered themselves obsolete they will merge as a prelude to their radical restructuring or abolition. The right population level for commissioning strategic regional services is of the order of one to two million. Once primary care trusts have been established, this is the likely scale of health authorities. A total number of authorities of 40 or less will certainly lead to a reduction in the number of NHS Executive Regional Offices and possibly their absorption into the central Executive. These changes could well occur early in the next Parliament or even sooner if primary care trusts are set up early.

Risks of change

All reorganizations have their risks and this is no exception. Denial, very possibly genuine, of the existence of a deliberate restructuring and, therefore, no blueprint, increases the risk. The basic rule is that local and small organizations can be flexible and sensitive but carry higher levels of risk. The proposals for primary care groups are typical of this genre; strong on community contact but weak on control and vulnerable to financial instability. In the past, higher bodies (regional health authorities) acted as the safety valve but it is unlikely that health authorities will have the power or resources to fulfil that role now. Mergers at all levels to reduce risk seems likely.

Changes in style and power

The impact of style

Language and style differentiate between societies and the sudden changes in language and corporate and individual behaviour which were heralded by the 1989 White Paper have exerted the most powerful impact on the health professions and their managers throughout the 1990s. Now the language is changing again and the corporate behaviour is going to change too; it is truly a new NHS. Of fundamental importance is the behaviour of Health Ministers and the way they treat key groups within the NHS. The continued recognition of primary care as central to the future of the NHS, the renewed involvement of clinicians in health service planning, a consistent and substantial boost for the nursing profession in national, local and primary care structures and even some less heated words for managers have sent positive signals to staff. Conversely, the economically necessary phasing of pay awards has dealt a severe blow to the popularity of the Government with NHS staff, although annual pay is a short-term issue and the actual level of awards for 1998/99 is quite generous. The unashamed abolition of fundholding and the construction of primary care groups which do not match existing GP commissioning groupings are blows to the majority of the GP community. Furthermore, the attitude of Ministers to the rare but inevitable disasters in health and social care have been concerned with attributing blame rather than seeking long-term solutions to intractable problems. On balance, therefore, there are very mixed messages coming from Ministers. They expect results and will not tolerate failure but they are likely to reward success and to remain loyal to those who behave as their friends.

Ever-changing power structures

The previous reforms induced the most radical shift in professional power structures for almost a century – managers became more important than doctors; general practitioners were in the ascendant over consultants; the number of nurses in primary care soared, though their status may not have risen much and they remain employees of the owners (GPs); counsellors emerged from nowhere; other new disciplines were created, such as clinical audit; executive directors became members of NHS trusts and health authority boards. There is no doubt that these new proposals will change the power structures again. In the ascendant are consultants and nurses of all types and in the opposite direction go managers and individual general practices. The long-term impact of these changes is difficult to predict. Professions have been given a boost before, only to be found wanting in terms of their capacity to take advantage of the opportunity (public health medicine is an example). The key opportunity now belongs to nursing. The Government clearly feels that nurses can change the balance of power between health care and the community as a whole. There is evidence that nurses are more sensitive to patients' needs and that they are closer in empathy to patients than doctors are ever likely to be. There are, however, indications that the public is falling out of love with nurses and there are growing numbers of reports of appalling practice, almost always in hospitals and usually involving the care of elderly people. Lack of cleanliness, caring and attention are the main criticisms, and the usual excuse of lack of resources is outrageous; it does not require an increase in taxes to avoid laziness, slovenliness and incompetence. The nursing profession has been exceptionally loyal to Labour through the last three decades and it may well be considered that it is time to repay the debt. For the NHS, the main battleground is in primary care where nurses are poised to become the largest profession but, traditionally and structurally, have none of the power. By giving community nursing a power base in each primary care group, there is a real chance that the professional managers and leaders of at least some of these groups will be nurses. It will follow in due course that general practitioners of the future will be employed by primary care trusts which are headed by professional nurses. The importance of such a change would not just be to promote nurses and nursing but the decline in power and authority of doctors who, through the partnership structure, actually own primary care.

Future funding of the NHS and health and social care

The general scene

Health care costs are rising throughout the world. The rise in the UK has been lower and slower than in many comparable countries but it has still been sufficient to embarrass successive governments. The reasons for rising costs are extensive (*see* Box 27) and are unlikely to be reversed by government action or any other event.

Box 27   The causes of rising health costs

- Ageing of the population

- Advancing medical and pharmaceutical technology

- Prolonged survival of people with chronic disease

- Rising public expectations for advanced treatments

- Reducing ageism and sexism in health care

- Increasing standards in professional practice

- Rising real costs through pay and price inflation

- Long-term survival of children with severe disability

While most governments in the developed world struggle to limit the pace of growth in health care costs, the battle appears destined to be lost regardless of the endeavour, commitment, pain endured and friends lost. The record in the UK is as good as anywhere and is attributed mainly to the near monopoly of the government-funded NHS and the use of cash limits and general management to control expenditure. No other system in the world comes as close to financial balance. The problem for the UK is that almost all the growth in health care costs is borne by the NHS, the private sector being unusually small and focused on the niche market of elective surgery. If health care costs continue to rise, as they undoubtedly will, the issue is whether the costs will be met from general taxation in the usual way the NHS is funded or whether an alternative funding system is adopted, such as mutual insurance or co-payments (a system where patients pay for part of the cost of their care). Successive investigations into NHS funding have continually reported that the existing funding mechanism is the most economic both for the Government and for the country as a whole.

The medium-term prospect for funding

The Government has rejected the notion that the funding of the NHS is so compromised that fundamental change is necessary. This is not to suggest that more money is not required; it assumes both that some resources can be released from existing services by improving efficiency and that the funding deficiency is at worst modest and manageable with steady annual increases. The Government has committed itself to increase funding each year and its initial actions have been consistent with a more generous outlook for the NHS than its recent history. Public sector finances are in a better state now than for a decade with the probability of a budget surplus at the end of the millennium. It is therefore likely that growth in NHS funding over the medium term will be at least 2% in real terms and that this will prove sufficient to keep it relatively secure and enable significant improvements in services, especially waiting time reductions. However, there is a genuine risk of much of this increase being swallowed up in pay rises for lower paid staff, especially if the minimum wage is set above £3.50 per hour. There is also the prospect of a sharp short-term boost for funding arising from the comprehensive spending review. This will result in a shift in total government funding from other departments to health and education and could be very substantial. The Government's anxiety to meet its election promise to cut waiting list numbers by 100000 has already resulted in an unexpected additional £500 million bonus for the NHS in 1998 as an advance payment on up to £3 billion during the life of this parliament.

The longer-term funding scenario

The global health care funding crisis will continue unabated for the foreseeable future. It is possible, but unlikely, that the existing funding mechanisms can continue. It is more likely that all the existing trends in costs will continue to rise with increasing speed and the health systems in most countries will either collapse or bankrupt the governments. In the UK, such a catastrophe is less likely as relative expenditure is low and the gap between income and expenditure is marginal. Nonetheless, the pressures experienced by the NHS during the last three years are likely to recur and governments will seek alternative solutions to the obvious one: spending a greater proportion of tax income on health care.

The recently established Royal Commission on long-term care could well hold the key to the future of the welfare state. Security and financial comfort in old age is vital to the future of our ageing and increasingly disabled population. At the lower end of the age range, more success in education holds the key to improving health under the age of 65. In older people, reduction in poverty is vital to maintaining health. Both lie at the heart of the Government's overarching strategy to deal with social exclusion. Success in this venture would do more for health than increasing expenditure on the NHS.

Allocation and distribution

Since regional health authorities were abolished, NHS resources have been allocated direct to district health authorities. These allocations, and those before them to regional and district health authorities since 1977, have been based on moving towards target allocations based on fair shares of the total budget. The formula on which these targets are based changes from time to time, usually in keeping with the political priorities of the day. Thus, changes in the formula have been used to protect teaching hospitals, to protect London, to protect all inner cities and to compensate rural areas. The current formula is based on a combination of census variables which together allow for standard utilization of services. It is poised to change again in a way which gives more resource to the most deprived areas. This redistribution will focus not on the funds for hospital and community health services, which have been the only funds affected by earlier formulae, but on the funding of primary care, especially general medical services. The maldistribution of these resources is at least twice as inequitable as those for hospitals.

Once the new structures are established, it is possible that allocations will be made direct to primary care groups. It will be for health authorities to decide how and whether to earmark resources for specific sectors of the service and to decide the speed with which primary care groups move towards their share of the target allocation. This allocation responsibility will be one of the main levers which health authorities will have to exert over primary care groups and a key tool in reducing inequalities.

The future relationship between the NHS and local authority social services

Local government and health

For most of modern times, local authorities led the campaign against ill health, initially through civil engineering (clean water and safe sewerage), workplace improvements, better housing and environmental hygiene, and later through the development of specialist hospitals (for infectious diseases and tuberculosis) and general hospitals. By 1926, most of the nation's health care was in the hands of local authorities – albeit financially supported from voluntary and central funds – and it remained there until 1948. The nationalization of the hospitals under the terms of the *NHS Act* left local authorities with limited responsibilities for public health and community nursing services, together with a range of developing social care services including old people's homes. In 1974, these responsibilities were split, health and health care transferring to the new NHS health authorities and the remainder forming (in 1972) new and growing social services departments in local authorities. Continued local authority involvement in health was restricted to food safety and hygiene and joint planning for those client groups which involved their own services (children, elderly, disabled, mentally ill and learning disabilities). These arrangements have continued to the present day with varying degrees of success. However, the boundary between health care and the ever-growing social care has been acknowledged as one of the major obstacles to high-quality care, as great a problem as the divisions within health care itself. Local authorities do not have health care responsibilities and, as described earlier, most counsellors resist involvement in issues which are beyond their financial responsibility with the exception of campaigns against so-called quangos (quasi-autonomous non-governmental organizations such as health authorities and NHS trusts). They are, indeed, restricted from spending their money on activities which are outwith their statutory duties beyond certain limits. Few counsellors have any experience of health services except as patients or if they are NHS staff themselves.

Joint planning

The post-1974 reorganization arrangements left in place joint responsibilities for planning care group services and provided hypothecated NHS funds to promote joint service developments, so-called joint finance. The existence of these resources effectively stifled joint service planning as it became an annual spending exercise and restricted long-term plans for rapidly expanding needs of the care groups concerned. The current proposals extend the principles of joint planning to embrace primary and community health care and social care together with specialist health care through service commissioning. The engagement of local authorities in this process, via the Health Improvement Programmes, is mandatory but does not give them a lead role. This must be considered as a deliberate act and not an oversight; the implications for local authority leadership in this field under the present Government are not good. Instead, it appears as if health authorities are to be the lead agency for planning adult services across all existing boundaries and primary care trusts will constitute the framework for integrated service provision. Local authorities are expected to deliver but health authorities must lead. It appears likely either that the existing rules for the use of joint finance and for resource transfer between authorities will be relaxed, and possibly the resource extended, in order to facilitate the development of new relationships, or that the whole system will be abolished and that primary care trusts will be required to commission or provide services across care sector boundaries in order to secure continuity of care.

Accountability

The unnerving reality for health and local authorities can be summed up thus; health authorities will be held to account for the performance of local authorities over whom they have no structural, moral or financial control and against whom they have no sanctions to exert. The price of failure to deliver by the local authorities and their performance will be a wholly undesirable visitation from CHIMP or the Audit Commission. This situation is analogous to the role of health authorities in respect of primary care; an unsustainable position which the primary care trust proposals acknowledge. How long will it be before the inconsistency of the above is recognized by a radical restructuring of the public sector? The future outlook for joint service accountability probably lies in devolution for England to the regions. The integration of health and local government cannot seriously be contemplated without some element of local democracy; the regional level is less risky than the existing framework of local government. Such a radical change will not occur during this Parliament but may be considered by Labour for a second term in office. Indeed, regional government in England has been an aspiration for prospective Labour government second terms since Margaret Thatcher abolished the Metropolitan Counties and the Greater London Council with effect from 1986.

Local authorities and primary care groups

For the first time in the history of the modern welfare system, local authorities will be directly involved in the governance of the whole NHS. Through their membership of primary care groups, they will have an influence over primary care for the first time. As well as ensuring that there is public involvement in primary care groups, local authority involvement will begin to establish a public mandate for the management of primary care and for the other functions of primary care groups/trusts.

The public health Green Paper: *Our Healthier Nation*

A new type of contract

Having eventually released its Green Paper on public health, the Government can be quietly pleased with its reception. Compared with its predecessor, *Health of the Nation*, the Green Paper has a much tighter focus, a more open approach to ownership, leadership and responsibility and, most important of all, a recognition of the vital inter-relationship between poverty and ill health. *Our Healthier Nation* is a consultation document on which views are sought. It is, however, relatively mature in its conception and the shape of the national strategy for health is already clearly visible. With a consultation period of less than three months and publication of the subsequent White Paper to follow shortly afterwards, the die is cast.

In addition to clearly stated aims (*see* Box 28) and targets (*see* Box 29), the basic currency of the strategy is a set of tripartite contracts between the Government, management agencies (such as health authorities, local authorities, schools or employers) and the people. The contract is outlined for the strategy as a whole, for each target and for each of three key settings in which action is required: schools – for children; workplaces – for adults; and neighbourhoods – for elderly people.

Box 28   The Government's key aims in *Our Healthier Nation*

- To improve the health of the population as a whole by increasing the length of people's lives and the number of years people spend free from illness

- To improve the health of the worst off in society and to narrow the health gap

---

Box 29   National health targets in *Our Healthier Nation*

By the year 2010 (baseline year the average of 1996, 1997 and 1998):

- **Heart disease and stroke** – to reduce the death rate from heart disease and stroke and related illnesses among people aged under 65 years by at least **a third**

- **Accidents** – to reduce accidents by at least **a fifth**

- **Cancer** – to reduce the death rate from cancer among people aged under 65 years by at least **a fifth**

- **Mental health** – to reduce the death rate from suicide and undetermined injury by **a sixth**

These are interesting policies, representing major changes in strategy and approach to the health of the population. It would be wrong and grossly unfair to criticize the previous Government for *Health of the Nation*, flawed though it was, as it constituted the first attempt in modern times to focus attention on population level health gain. *Our Healthier Nation* should be seen as improving and redirecting the national strategy for health; the special character-istics being a focus on preventing premature death (under the age of retirement at 65), reducing inequalities in health and reducing the duration of illness and disability. Only the first of these is likely to be achieved but there will be a good deal of attention on the attempts to pursue the others and success is not out of the question.

Moving targets

Although there are superficial similarities between the new targets and the old, there are more profound and important differences. The key areas are the same except for the dropping of sexual health which is to be addressed in a separate policy. The new targets for reducing death rates focus on cardiovascular disease and stroke and cancer in under 65-year-olds for whom they account for two-thirds of all deaths. The far more numerous deaths in 65–74-year-old people which featured in *Health of the Nation* have been dropped. It could be argued that they were chosen simply for the sake of it without any clear goal other than measurement, whereas the new target, backed by the drive on inequalities, sets out to achieve an increase in survivors beyond working age, to enjoy the fruits of retirement. The behavioural targets in *Health of the Nation* have also been dropped, mainly because they were unattainable but also because they were pointless, it being health outcomes that constituted their purpose. The greatest weakness of the previous Government's strategy was their unwillingness to take action to support their own targets, especially in tobacco and alcohol consumption. The new Government remains 'on approval' in this regard but a White Paper or the equivalent on tobacco control is planned for later in 1998. The target for accidents replaces several targets focused on different age groups; the new target is to reduce accidents themselves rather than deaths from accidents as previously. Accidents in children and in elderly people display very high class differentials; reducing these excesses in poor people would be a prime example of success in the fight against social exclusion. Accidental deaths in young adults, a *Health of the Nation* target, reflect car usership and are more common in affluent and rural settings. The least robust, and most disappointing, target – and therefore likely to come in for most criticism – is that for suicide. The targeting of suicide assumes that suicide is wrong and avoidable, that it can be prevented by health service and other community action and that it can be reliably measured. In fact, suicide can be a rational action by a distressed but not mentally ill person; unlike observations in the 1960s, most suicides, especially young men (the group causing most concern) do not seek medical help shortly before the act and Coroner's Court verdicts can appear to be based on the interests of the family rather than the facts.

Factor analysis

The Green Paper will be widely used by students as a source for statistics on health inequalities and trends in health performance. It is rather surprising that so few copies were made available to the NHS; the whole paper is available on the Internet but the graphs and figures do not download well and the original in colour is required to make presentations. It also includes an intelligent analysis of the factors which affect health (*see* Box 30). Special attention is given to the impact of unemployment on early death, the consequences of smoking, ethnicity and social class variations.

Box 30   Factors affecting health

- *Fixed*
  1 Genes
  2 Sex
  3 Ageing

- *Social and economic*
  1 Poverty
  2 Employment
  3 Social exclusion

- *Environment*
  1 Air quality
  2 Housing
  3 Water quality
  4 Social environment

- *Lifestyle*
  1 Diet
  2 Physical activity
  3 Smoking
  4 Alcohol
  5 Sexual behaviour
  6 Drugs

- *Access to services*
  1 Education
  2 NHS
  3 Social services
  4 Transport
  5 Leisure

Contracts for health

The scene is set for the Green Paper by the overall contract for health. There is also a contract for each of the four priority areas and for each setting. For each contract, the possible actions of the Government are listed alongside those for local organizations and for the relevant group of people. Typical examples are given in Box 31.

Box 31   Examples of the national contracts

A contract for health

- *Government*
  Tackle the root causes of ill health

- *Local players*
  Plan and provide high-quality services to everyone who needs them

- *People*
  Take responsibility for their own health and make healthier choices about their lifestyle

Healthy schools

- *Government*
  Set high educational standards

- *Schools*
  Give children the capacity to make the most of their lives and their future families' lives

- *Pupils and parents*
  Work together to share responsibility for academic achievement, healthier eating, better exercise and a responsible attitude to smoking, drugs, alcohol, sex and relationships

Healthy workplaces

- *Government*
  Ensure minimum employment rights to encourage decent and responsible partnerships between staff and managers

---

- *Employers*
  Take measures to reduce stress at work

- *Employees*
  Support colleagues who have problems or who are disabled

The national contracts for the four priority areas cover four discrete factors as well as the three constituencies for action. These factors are social and economic, environmental, lifestyle and services. An example for heart disease and stroke is shown in Box 32.

Box 32 Examples of action to help achieve the target for heart disease and stroke

A national contract on heart disease and stroke	Government and national players can:	Local players and communities can:	People can:
Social and economic	Continue to make smoking cost more through taxation.	Provide incentives to employees to cycle or walk to work, or leave their cars at home.	Take opportunities to better their lives through education, training and employment.
Environmental	Encourage employers to provide a smoke-free environment for non-smokers.	Through local employers and staff, work in partnership to reduce stress at work.	Protect others from second-hand smoke.
Lifestyle	End advertising and promotion of cigarettes.	Encourage the development of healthy schools and healthy workplaces.	Stop smoking or cut down, watch what they eat and take regular exercise.
Services	Encourage doctors and nurses to give advice on healthier living.	Provide help to people who want to stop smoking.	Have their blood pressure checked regularly.

Local choices

In addition to the four national priority areas, Health Improvement Programmes are expected to include a limited range of additional local priorities reflecting local communities and the issues which concern them. The Green Paper suggests some local priorities (*see* Box 33) which will no doubt be added to and refined during the consultation period.

Box 33   Possible local priorities and targets

- Asthma and other respiratory problems

- Teenage pregnancy

- Infant mortality

- Back pain, rheumatism and arthritis

- Environment

- Diabetes

- Oral health

- Vulnerable groups

Final thoughts

Our Healthier Nation is destined to become an enigma. The flaws in the process of its introduction, and the impression the paper gives that it was written by a committee, detracts from its many strengths. It describes the problems of inequality in the context of steady overall improvements in health (in general) and places a clear focus on where, how and by whom improvements need to be made. It is, perhaps, a little idealistic in terms of the language of the contract; it is far more likely that the public expects the Government to fulfil its part of the bargain, than the Government expects the public to fulfil its side. Nonetheless, as a consultation paper, with time during 1998 to clarify its focus and targets, it provides a sound basis for the improvements in the health of the community which the affluence of the millennium ought to deliver for the whole community.

A world of paradox

In finalizing this review of the new Government's policies on health and the NHS, I am struck by the omnipresence of paradox in modern society. The sometimes strained relationship between government and the people is the embodiment of a combination of desires to be led and to be free. The complex inter-relationships between wealth, health, education, behaviour, demand, need and supply and the inevitability of inequality in any society true to itself, makes our world impossible to manage from a central point. Creating the right context and passing the right laws are the roles of central government. The greatest gap in our political system is a model of local democracy which can address local aspects of national issues. This is what devolution offers to Scotland and the same principles should be applied to the English regions if local ownership of the management of public services is to be conducted in a discernible democratic framework. There are those who will proclaim that democracy does not work in a modern society because the issues and networks are too complex. I would respond that any other system is worse and, anyway, true democracy has not really been tested yet. This is why the devolution experiment is so important. For once, the Scots want to pilot a model of political management which might provide the answer to England's problems.

Further reading

Department of Health (1998) *The New NHS: modern, dependable. A National Framework for Assessing Performance*. Consultation document, EL(98)4. Department of Health, Leeds.
Department of Health (1998) *Our Healthier Nation: a contract for health*. Department of Health, London.

Department of Health (1998) *National Service Frameworks*. HSC 1998 (074). Department of Health, London.

Department of Health (1998) *The New NHS: commissioning specialised services*. Consultation document. Department of Health, London.

Department of Health (1998) *The New NHS: modern, dependable. Establishing Primary Care Groups*. HSC 1998 (065). Department of Health, London.

Department of Health (1997) *The New NHS: modern, dependable*. Department of Health, London.

Department of Health (1997) *Health Action Zones: invitations to bid*. EL(97)65. Department of Health, London.

Audit Commission (1997) *Higher Purchase: commissioning specialised services in the NHS*. Audit Commission, London.

Department of Health (1995) *Commissioning Cancer Services – Report of the Expert Advisory Group on Cancer*. Department of Health, London (The Calman–Hine Report).

Department of Health (1989) *Working for Patients*. Department of Health, London.

Index